AF386627

Basic Principles of Epidemiology

This book is an up-to-date, user-friendly textbook that aims to make epidemiological methods easy to learn and apply in public health research. Written in clear and accessible language, the book simplifies complex topics for easy understanding with examples, making it ideal for students, researchers, and public health professionals at all levels – from undergraduates to postgraduates and educators.

The book has a unique combination of relevance, comprehensive coverage, and practical explanations to provide students with a thorough grounding in key epidemiological concepts and methods such as study designs, measures of association, evaluation of a diagnostic test, bias, confounding and interaction, and more.

- Easy to read and understand, with practical examples to explain key concepts.
- Provides essential epidemiological concepts and methods, making it most suitable for beginners, intermediate students, and practicing epidemiologists in medical and public health studies and research.
- Includes chapters that are often overlooked in other epidemiology books, such as measures of agreement, sample size calculation, sampling methods, and the application of AI in public health.

Beyond standard topics, the book includes essential yet often overlooked chapters such as measures of agreement, sample size calculations, sampling methods, and the application of AI in public health, equipping readers with skills that are vital in modern research and practice.

Easy to read, the book is an invaluable resource for beginners and intermediate students and practicing epidemiologists who play an active role in medical and public health studies and research.

Basic Principles of Epidemiology

Second Edition

Mohammad Tajul Islam
MBBS, DTM&H, MSc (CTM), MPH
Adjunct Faculty, Department of Public Health
North South University, Bangladesh
Former Technical Advisor, JICA and
Senior Advisor, Save the Children

Mohammad Delwer Hossain Hawlader
MBBS, MPH, PhD
Professor, Department of Public Health and
Director, NSU Global Health Institute (NGHI)
North South University, Bangladesh

Russell Kabir
BDS, MPH, MSc, PhD
Associate Professor of Public Health & Biostatistics
School of Allied Health and Social Care
Faculty of Health, Medicine and Social Care
Anglia Ruskin University, Essex, UK

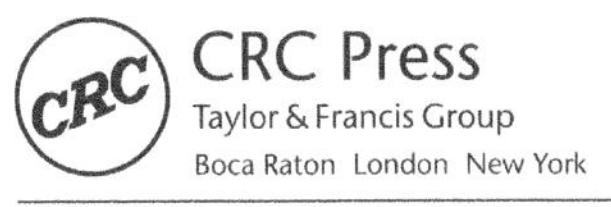

CRC Press
Taylor & Francis Group
Boca Raton London New York

CRC Press is an imprint of the
Taylor & Francis Group, an **informa** business

A CHAPMAN & HALL BOOK

Designed cover image: Shutterstock

Second edition published 2026
by CRC Press
2385 NW Executive Center Drive, Suite 320, Boca Raton FL 33431

and by CRC Press
4 Park Square, Milton Park, Abingdon, Oxon, OX14 4RN

CRC Press is an imprint of Taylor & Francis Group, LLC

© 2026 Mohammad Tajul Islam, Mohammad Delwer Hossain Hawlader, and Russell Kabir

First edition published by ASA Publishing Corporation 2023

First edition published by ASA Publications 2023

ISBN: 9781041101772 (hbk)
ISBN: 9781041103936 (pbk)
ISBN: 9781003654803 (ebk)

DOI: 10.1201/9781003654803

Typeset in Palatino
by Newgen Publishing UK

Contents

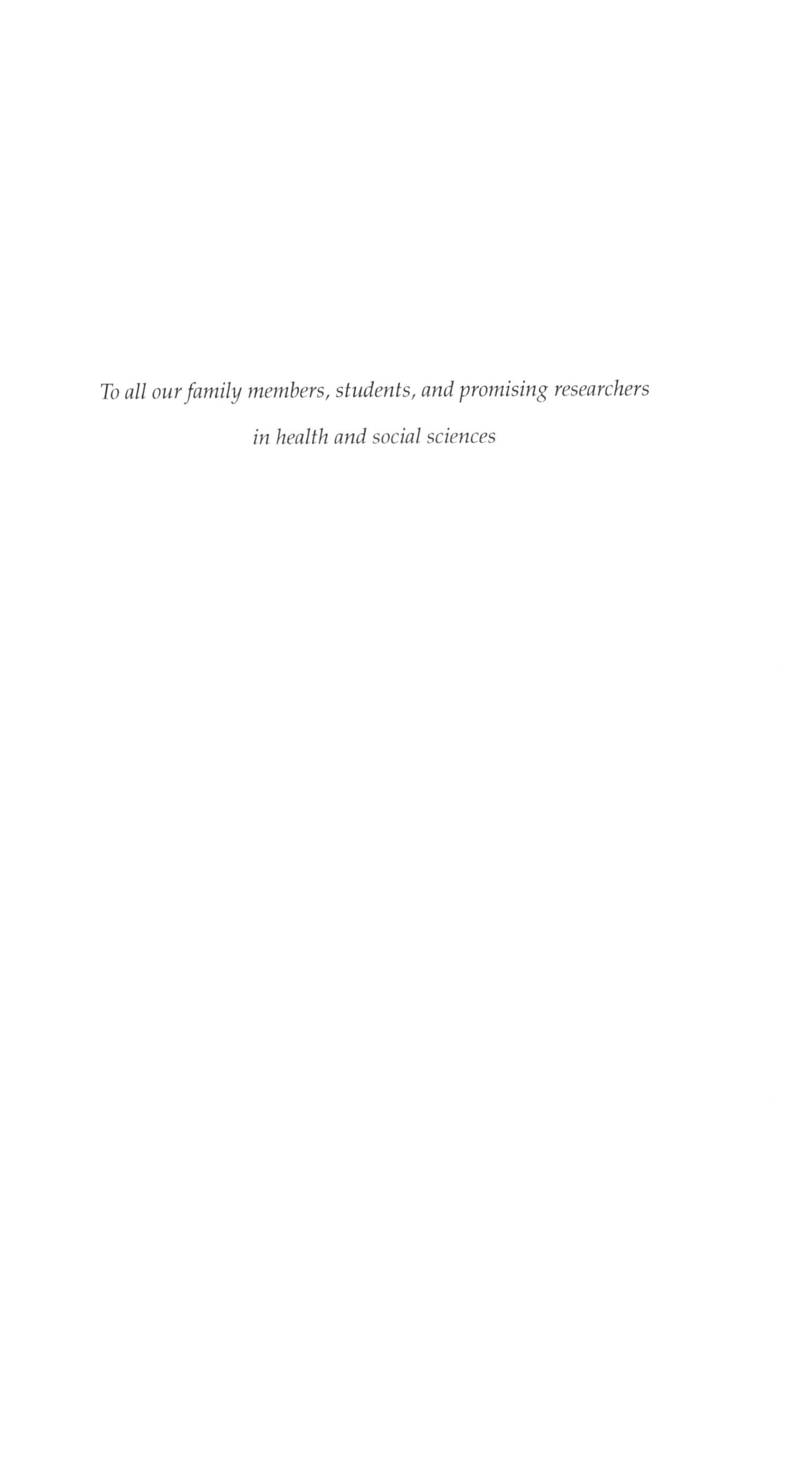

To all our family members, students, and promising researchers

in health and social sciences

Foreword

It was a pleasure writing a foreword to this book. As a medical student, when I was learning epidemiology nearly 35 years ago, there were limited suitable reference books to guide junior doctors and public health researchers like me. That all began to change since then, and we had a plethora of books and guidance or journal papers to consider when deciding on something to recommend to the students at every level, from beginners to advanced postgraduates.

The authors of the current book have given much thought to creating a user-friendly reference book that guides readers throughout their journey in the epidemiology world. They are long-standing experts in health service and social science research methods – the reader is in good hands. It is worth having a look at some of their published books and academic papers utilizing population-level data to understand and improve public health provision globally; all of these research outputs have been established based on their strong knowledge and skills in epidemiology.

The aim of the book is to make the understanding of epidemiology easy and explicit. I am sure this book would be a handy companion reference to students and early-career researchers in population health. One of the distinctive features of this book from all the others could be the clarity of the concepts and approaches introduced to the essential aspects of practical epidemiology. It explains the fundamental concepts in a simple, digestible format with an example. Therefore, this is instrumental for further epidemiology practice by public health practitioners, junior health services researchers, and university students using the latest statistical packages to analyze data and properly interpret them.

It had been a privilege to receive and read the book. I personally know their works and have a high regard for the authors of the chapters. This textbook guides us through properly selected population health analysis and interpretations, reducing room for error while helping to build confidence through practice. The book has a logical framework and structure, proceeding from sections on concepts and methods to statistical methods to applications and fields of current research. I enjoyed reading these accounts, and I am confident that many others will do so too.

As an academic who has taught population health subjects including epidemiology modules (basic and advanced) over the last 25 years, very often I observed that some students were able to run the statistical analysis using software packages (e.g., SPSS) but struggled to properly absorb the results or do the basic analysis manually. I am confident that this book sits next to the most preferred key textbooks that students and researchers enjoy returning to whenever they struggle to understand statistical analysis of outputs, or if they want to check the interpretations suggesting decisions or policies at the population health level themselves.

Finally, I am obliged to mention that the authors have devoted a considerable amount of time to writing this book. **All profits from sales will be donated to their chosen charities in support of good causes.** I am sure you will appreciate their intention and generosity and would recommend reading the book.

Dr. Ali Davod Parsa
MD (GP), PhD (Health Economist), PGDip (HSR), PGCE, PGCBA
FRSPH, FHEA, FIHM, FCMI, M-SSM, M-EUPHA
Associate Professor of Health Economics, Policy, and Management
Public Health Course and Modules Leader
Former Advisor, Deputy Cabinet Minister of Health in Medical Education, Iran
Faculty of Health, Medicine, and Social Care
Anglia Ruskin University, Cambridge, UK

Preface

Inspired by the positive reception of our first edition and the valuable feedback from readers and students, we present the updated second edition of the book. The purpose of this book remains to present the basic concepts and methods of epidemiology as they are applied to disease or health-related problem investigation and intervention designs in an understandable manner.

In this edition, we have introduced new chapters on important topics, such as standardization of rates, measures of agreement, Type I and Type II errors, sampling methods, and application of artificial intelligence (AI) in public health. These additions will provide readers with a deeper understanding of essential epidemiological techniques. Additionally, we have thoroughly reviewed and revised the content of existing chapters to ensure clarity, relevance, and alignment with contemporary practices. As with the previous edition, we have maintained our approach of providing concise yet comprehensive explanations, with references to additional resources to explore specific topics in more detail.

Designed primarily for introductory courses in epidemiology at the undergraduate and graduate levels, this book serves a wide audience of students (e.g., MPH, MSc, MS, MD, FCPS, MPhil, and PhD) and professionals in public health, medicine, dentistry, veterinary medicine, and social sciences. Teachers, researchers, and public health practitioners will also find it a valuable resource for building a foundational understanding of epidemiological principles and methods.

The ongoing evolution of public health challenges, with the emergence of new diseases and the reemergence of old ones, heightens the growing need for skilled epidemiologists in preventive medicine and research. We hope this updated edition will continue to meet the needs of students and professionals, providing a solid grounding in the principles of epidemiology and helping them to step up into more advanced studies in epidemiology. For readers interested in statistical data analysis, we also recommend our books "Learning SPSS without Pain (ASA Publications, 2021)" and "Data Analysis with Stata (ASA Publications, 2022)".

As always, we welcome feedback and suggestions from our readers, which will help us further improve future editions of this book.

M. Tajul Islam

Acknowledgments

We are grateful to Mr. Md. Golam Kibria, Dr. SM Anwar Sadat, and Mr. Zunayed Al Azdi, who reviewed this book and provided their critical views and constructive suggestions. We are particularly thankful to Dr. Ali Davod Parsa for his careful review and for writing the foreword for this book. We are indebted to Mr. Zariath Al-Mamun Badhon and Mr. Md. Nazmul Hasan for their contributions in typesetting.

We would like to acknowledge and thank our well-wishers, Mrs. Madhini Sivasubramanian of University of Sunderland, London, UK; Dr. Haniya Zehra Syed and Dr. Richard Hayhoe of Anglia Ruskin University, UK; Prof. Hafiz T. A. Khan of University of West London, UK; Dr. S. M. Yasir Arafat of Enam Medical College & Hospital, Dhaka, Bangladesh; Dr. Fahima Nasrin Eva of North South University, Bangladesh; Dr. Mosharraf Sarker of Liverpool John Moores University, Liverpool, UK; and Dr. Rajeeb Kumar Sah of University of Huddersfield, Huddersfield, UK, for their continued support and valuable suggestions.

Many of our students and academics, who continually pushed and encouraged us to write this book, deserve a share of the credit, including Dr. Shakil Ahmed and Dr. Al-Afroza Sultana. We, the authors, accept full responsibility for any deficiencies or errors that the book may have. Finally, we express our sincerest thanks to Taylor & Francis for publishing this book.

1

Introduction

Russell Kabir

People around the world are living longer due to a significant reduction in early deaths because of effective preventive measures, improvements, and accessibility to health care services, improved nutrition, safe water supplies, better sanitation, and more. However, this increase in lifespan has led to a rise in disease burden. Disease patterns are also changing with the emergence of new diseases.

Public health focuses on protecting and improving the health of populations by identifying the distribution and causes of diseases or health-related problems and by preventing and responding to them. Research is an integral part of public health, helping to identify the causes of health problems and providing suggestions for interventions. Epidemiology, the science of investigating the occurrence of diseases in the community and determining their causes through systematic data collection and analysis, plays a crucial role in this process.

1.1 Definition of Epidemiology

In his 1978 seminal paper, Lilienfeld defined epidemiology as a "method of reasoning about a disease that deals with biological inference derived from observations of disease phenomena in a population group" [1]. In 1979, Evans defined epidemiology as "the quantitative analysis of the circumstances under which disease processes, including trauma, occur in population groups, the factors affecting their incidence, distribution and host responses and the use of knowledge in prevention and control" [2].

Vaughan et al. (1991) defined epidemiology as "the study of the distribution of problems related to health and disease and their determinants in human populations. Epidemiology aims to collect, interpret, and use information to promote health and reduce disease" [3]. The most popular definition of epidemiology that is commonly used is given by Last (2004): *"The study of distribution and determinants of health-related states or events in specified populations and the application of this study to control health problems"* [4].

DOI: 10.1201/9781003654803-1

Epidemiology deals with individuals belonging to a particular group and having specific characteristics. Epidemiology deals with the population. When we look at the epidemiology of a specific health condition, health problem, or disease, we look at its distribution and determinants. The distribution of a disease in a population can be described in terms of person, place, and time. We try to understand who is affected by that health condition, where it is happening, and when. Knowing the descriptive epidemiology of a particular disease helps us better plan for efficiently allocating resources to control that disease.

In addition to describing a particular health problem, epidemiology also investigates or analyzes the determinants (factors associated with) of that disease condition. The determinants could be risk factors or protective factors. Risk factors are associated with an increased likelihood of the occurrence of a particular disease or its consequences in each population, e.g., smoking is associated with different types of cancer (lung cancer, oral cancer, and others). The protective factors are the factors that are associated with a reduced likelihood of disease occurrence, such as vaccination against disease. Analytic epidemiology helps us plan to investigate the factors associated with a disease and decide on interventions.

In brief, epidemiology generates evidence based on which health professionals and policymakers design programs and implement them to promote the health of a particular population. And this is precisely where it is linked to public health.

Example

Tuberculosis (TB) is a major public health problem in Bangladesh. To control tuberculosis, in terms of both prevention and treatment, a sound understanding of the epidemiology of TB in Bangladesh is essential. A study was conducted in the Matlab sub-district of Bangladesh in 2001 to estimate the prevalence of TB in a rural population aged 15 years or above [5]. If the sputum of a suspected case of TB (defined as having a cough for more than three weeks) was positive for acid-fast bacilli (AFB), that person was considered a case of TB. Table 1.1 shows the distribution of TB cases by age and gender [5]. The prevalence of TB was significantly higher among males than among females. Clustering was identified while looking at the geographical distribution of TB cases (Figure 1.1).

1.2 Uses of Epidemiology

Epidemiology helps to:

- Identify the causative factors or agents for a disease or health events by observation or experiment.

TABLE 1.1

Age and gender distribution of AFB-positive cases

Age (years)	Sex					
	Male		Female		Total	
	Tested	Sputum positive (%)	Tested	Sputum positive (%)	Tested	Sputum positive (%)
15-24	203	3 (1.5)	191	3 (1.6)	394	6 (1.5)
25-34	230	5 (2.2)	282	1 (0.4)	512	6 (1.2)
35-44	365	9 (2.5)	392	2 (0.5)	757	11 (1.5)
>45	1249	25 (2.0)	922	4 (0.4)	2171	29 (1.3)
All	2047	42 (2.1)*	1787	10 (0.6) *	3834	52 (1.4)

AFB, Acid-fast bacillus
* $P<0.001$

Source: Matlab, 2001. Data from Ref. [5].

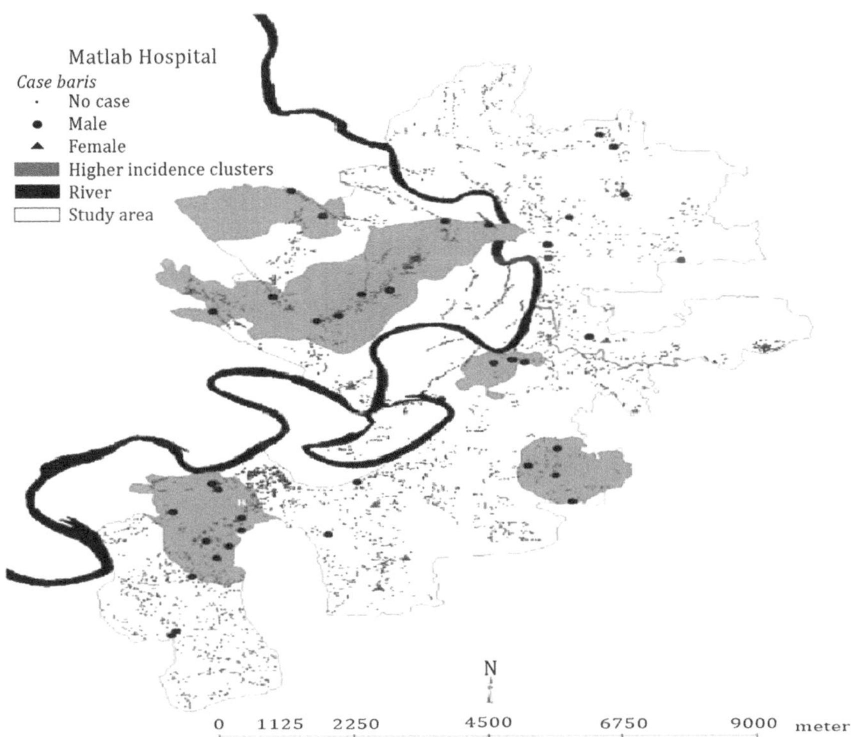

FIGURE 1.1

Geographic clusters of increased risk of TB, Matlab study area. (Ref. [5])

- Observe the natural history and outcome of the disease by explaining how and why the disease occurs.

- Estimating the burden of diseases in a population is a valuable tool for community diagnosis by assessing the presence, nature, and distribution of health and disease among the people.

- It can early estimate the factors that can put people at risk of disease and develop strategies to prevent or treat disease.

- Assessing the community's health needs and predicting future health needs.

- Epidemiological data is essential to plan, implement, and evaluate services for the prevention, control, and treatment of diseases, as well as to identify priorities to improve the health and well-being of people.

- Evaluate the effectiveness of health programs and formulate and implement public health policy and planning.

- Conduct surveillance of disease and health events occurrence in populations and of the risk factors [6–8].

1.3 Epidemiological Approaches

The approaches used in epidemiology include asking *questions and making comparisons.* Questions are asked to explore the health problem and its magnitude, areas and individuals affected by the disease, the time of occurrence, what actions have been taken, how the disease can be prevented in the future, and others. All these questions help identify disease etiologies and plan and evaluate interventions.

On the other hand, comparison is a basic approach in epidemiology. Comparisons are made to understand disease frequencies in different population groups, individual characteristics, geographical areas, and periods. Comparison helps the epidemiologist formulate and test hypotheses [9].

1.4 Scope of Epidemiology

Epidemiology, as an emerging science, has applications not only in the study of the occurrence of diseases or health problems in the population, but has also been effectively extended beyond the domain of health and disease conditions to other areas such as health-related events, healthcare and health services, population dynamics, psychological and behavioral science, accidents and injuries, evaluation of health intervention programs, health needs assessment of the community, and other branches of science and technology with an overarching goal to improve the health and wellbeing of the general population. The scopes of epidemiology are outlined below.

Causation of disease: The distribution of disease is described in terms of time, place, and person. Using different epidemiological study designs, hypotheses can be formulated, tested, and confirmed for disease causation. Different socioeconomic, genetic, and environmental factors are responsible for disease causation.

Natural history of disease: Epidemiology is very useful for understanding the natural history of a particular disease by exploring the agent, host, and environmental factors. The natural history of disease tells us how it advances from the earliest pre-pathogenesis stage to its cessation as recovery, disability, or death.

Health status of the population: With the help of epidemiology, public health professionals can easily assess the health status of a group of people in a particular setting or area. This will indicate the disease burden in the population and measures that can be taken to control or reduce the disease burden following epidemiological guidelines.

Classification of disease: Epidemiological investigation helps identify the determinants of disease; thus, the diseases can be classified according to the determinants. For example, Vibrio cholera bacteria is responsible for cholera infection, which is a communicable disease, and on the other hand, drinking too much alcohol for a prolonged period causes liver cirrhosis, which is a non-communicable disease. Based on the disease classification, further management of the disease is provided.

Mechanism of disease transmission: Epidemiology helps to understand the disease transmission mechanism. By stopping the disease's transmission, public health professionals can protect people from contracting the disease.

Evaluation of intervention: Epidemiological studies are used to evaluate the effectiveness of health services, planning, and health promotion programs, such as the efficiency of sanitation measures in controlling diarrheal disease.

Creating new evidence: Epidemiological evidence is based on scientific methods and concerns only evidence produced by quantitative methods. However, qualitative research methods are also crucial in epidemiology, primarily supporting and validating new epidemiological research findings [6, 10–13].

1.5 Essential Public Health Services

The essential public health services (EPHS) framework, created by the Public Health Functions Steering Committee, delineates public health systems' fundamental roles and duties. The EPHS framework includes ten fundamental services, categorized into three main functions: assessment, policy formulation, and assurance [14].

1.5.1 Assessment

The assessment process involves systematically collecting, analyzing, and disseminating information on the health of a community. This function includes two essential services:

> *Monitor Health Status to Identify and Solve Community Health Problems:* This service focuses on continuously gathering and examining data regarding health outcomes, risk factors, and healthcare access. Disease surveillance is an essential element, facilitating the timely identification of possible health risks [15]. Epidemiology is crucial to this service as it offers methods and tools for tracking disease patterns, spotting outbreaks, and evaluating population health risks [16]. For example, throughout the COVID-19 pandemic, epidemiological monitoring was vital for observing the virus's spread, recognizing high-risk populations, and assessing the efficacy of interventions [17].

> *Diagnose and Investigate Health Problems and Health Hazards in the Community:* This service emphasizes exploring the risk factors for diseases and detecting possible dangers in the community. Epidemiology plays a key role in carrying out outbreak investigations, pinpointing risk factors for illnesses, and assessing the effectiveness of interventions [15]. This entails applying epidemiological techniques to locate the origin of an outbreak, recognize the mode of transmission, and carry out control measures to halt further spread.

1.5.2 Policy Development

Policy development involves using scientific evidence and community input to develop policies and plans that support public health. This core function includes three essential services:

> *Inform, educate, and empower people about health issues:* This service focuses on communicating health information to the public and promoting healthy behaviors. Epidemiology contributes by providing data

on the prevalence of health problems, the effectiveness of interventions, and the risks associated with certain behaviors [15].

Mobilize community partnerships and action to identify and solve health problems: This service involves engaging community members and organizations to improve public health. Epidemiology can help identify community health needs and priorities and can also be used to evaluate the impact of community-based interventions [15].

Develop policies and plans that support individual and community health efforts: This service focuses on developing policies and plans that promote health and prevent disease. Epidemiology provides the evidence base for these policies and plans by identifying risk factors, evaluating the effectiveness of interventions, and projecting future health trends [15]. For example, epidemiological studies have been instrumental in informing tobacco control, vaccination, and food safety policies.

1.5.3 Assurance

Assurance ensures that essential health services are available and accessible to all community members. This core function includes five essential services:

Enforce laws and regulations that protect health and ensure safety: This service aims to uphold laws and regulations that safeguard public health, including food safety, water quality, and air pollution. Epidemiology supplies the information necessary to track adherence to these laws and regulations and to assess their efficacy in safeguarding public health [17].

Link people to needed personal health services and assure the provision of health care when otherwise unavailable: This service guarantees that all community members can access vital health services, such as primary care, mental health support, and treatment for substance abuse. Epidemiology can help identify populations with unmet health needs and can be used to evaluate the effectiveness of interventions designed to improve access to care [17].

Assure a competent public and personal healthcare workforce: This service focuses on ensuring the public health workforce has the knowledge and skills to address public health challenges effectively. Epidemiology training is essential for public health professionals, providing the tools to collect, analyze, interpret data, conduct research, and evaluate programs [17].

Evaluate effectiveness, accessibility, and quality of personal and population-based health services: This service focuses on evaluating the effectiveness, accessibility, and quality of health services. Epidemiology provides the methods and tools to assess the impact of health programs and policies on health outcomes [17].

Research for new insights and innovative solutions to health problems: This service emphasizes the importance of researching to advance public health knowledge and develop innovative solutions to health problems [17]. Epidemiology is a research-intensive field, and epidemiologists play a key role in conducting studies to identify new risk factors for disease, evaluate the effectiveness of interventions, and develop new strategies for preventing disease and promoting health.

1.6 Role of Epidemiology in Public Health

Epidemiology is the science that studies the patterns, causes and effects of health and disease conditions in a defined population. It is the cornerstone of public health and informs policy decisions and evidence-based practice by identifying risk factors for disease and targets for preventive healthcare.

The evidence that epidemiology generates helps us better understand a particular health problem and go for appropriate intervention. Knowing the distribution and determinants of disease frequency for a specific population better guides us for effective health promotion. Opting for public health interventions without knowing epidemiology may result in outcomes and impacts that do not achieve the targets. This might result in inefficient allocation and use of resources, which are always scarce and under the pressure of multiple priorities [18, 19].

Example
Women of the reproductive age group who had access to mass media, about 68% of them used antenatal care services during their pregnancy and for the participants who did not have access to mass media, only 43% of the women used the antenatal care services (Table 1.2) [20]. Timely and regular utilization

TABLE 1.2

Relationship between mass media access and utilization of antenatal care services (ANC)

	Received ANC		
	No	Yes	Total
Had access to mass media	390 (32%)	794 (68%)	1,184
Did not have access	89 (57%)	67 (43%)	156
Total	479 (35.7%)	861 (64.2%)	1,340

Source: Data from [20].

of antenatal care services is an important indicator of reducing maternal mortality. Using this data, public health professionals can target women of reproductive age groups to educate them more about the services, and more public health promotion campaigns about antenatal care through mass media will influence them to seek the services.

1.7 History of Epidemiology

The word "epidemiology" is derived from the Greek words "Epi", meaning "Upon", and "Demons", meaning "People", and "logos", meaning study, i.e., the study of people, and this was coined by Hippocrates in 460–370 BC. Hippocrates mentioned the importance of studying the place (where), time (when), and the people affected (who and how). He further explored how the environment is associated with the causation of human disease.

The Greeks and Romans identified the relationship between seasonal changes and disease onset. Malaria epidemiology started then, and drainage and control measures were initiated in Ancient Greece and Rome.

Health statistics were introduced in the 17th century by John Graunt in London. In 1662, John Graunt started recording the age, gender, reason for death, and where and when of the deceased person. This helped John record the number of deaths and causes each year.

Thomas Sydenham, an Oxford graduate, identified three levels of fevers in London – continued fevers, which are now typhoid and typhus, intermittent fever, which is malaria and smallpox (including measles) in the 1660s and 1670s.

Bernardino Ramazzini, from Italy, in 1692, explored the relationship between barometric readings and the source of the disease by observing the daily readings from people affected by typhoid fever.

In 1768, Edward Jenner discovered a better approach to preventing smallpox by introducing the first vaccine, and he was convinced that cowpox could protect against smallpox.

John Snow, considered the pioneer of modern epidemiology, commenced his epidemiological journey by examining the distribution of cholera by time, place, and persons in the Broad Street Wall, London district. In 1854, John hypothesized that cholera spread through contaminated water and recommended improving the water supply in that area to control the cholera outbreak.

Joseph Goldberger identified in 1915 that pellagra disease is a nutritional origin, and consuming more animal products in the diet helps prevent the disease [6, 9, 11, 21, 22].

References

1. Lilienfeld DE. Definitions of epidemiology. *Am J Epidemiol*. 1978;107(2):87–90.
2. Evans AS. Re: "Definitions of epidemiology". *Am J Epidemiol*. 1979;109(3):379–82.
3. Vaughan JP, Morrow RH, World Health Organization. *Manual of Epidemiology for District Health Management*. Geneva: WHO; 1989.
4. Last JM, International Epidemiological Association. *A Dictionary of Epidemiology*. 4th ed. New York: Oxford University Press; 2001.
5. Zaman K, Yunus M, Arifeen SE, Baqui AH, Sack DA, et al. Prevalence of sputum smear-positive tuberculosis in a rural area in Bangladesh. *Epidemiol Infect*. 2006;134(5):1052–9. doi:10.1017/S0950268806006099
6. Deepti SS. *Fundamentals of Epidemiology and Biostatistics*. New Delhi: CBS Publishers; 2014.
7. Van den Broeck J, Brestoff JR, Baum M. Definition and scope of epidemiology. In: Van den Broeck J, Brestoff JR, eds. *Epidemiology: Principles and Practical Guidelines*. Dordrecht: Springer; 2013:3–18.
8. Smith GD. The uses of epidemiology. *Int J Epidemiol*. 2001;30(5):1146–55. doi:10.1093/ije/30.5.1146
9. Park K. *Park's Textbook of Preventive and Social Medicine*. 19th ed. Jabalpur: Banarasidas Bhanot; 2005.
10. Macera CA, Shaffer R, Shaffer PM. *Introduction to Epidemiology: Distribution and Determinants of Disease*. New York: Cengage Learning; 2013.
11. Gordis L. *Epidemiology*. 5th ed. Philadelphia: Elsevier Health Sciences; 2013.
12. Van den Broeck J, Brestoff JR, Kaulfuss C. *Epidemiology: Principles and Practical Guidelines*. Dordrecht: Springer; 2013.
13. Olsen J, Christensen K, Murray J, Ekbom A. *An Introduction to Epidemiology for Health Professionals*. New York: Springer; 2010.
14. Montero JT, Terrillion A. *Reintegrating Health Care and Public Health*. Philadelphia: Lippincott Williams & Wilkins; 2013.
15. Alfehaid AFS. Disease surveillance and public health: How epidemiology informs action. Power Syst Technol. 2024.
16. Friis RH, Sellers TA. *Epidemiology for Public Health Practice*. 6th ed. Burlington: Jones & Bartlett Learning; 2020.
17. Somerville M, Kumaran K, Anderson R. *Public Health and Epidemiology at a Glance*. 2nd ed. Hoboken: Wiley; 2016.
18. Savitz DA, Poole C, Miller WC. Reassessing the role of epidemiology in public health. *Am J Public Health*. 1999;89(8):1158–61. doi:10.2105/AJPH.89.8.1158
19. Detels R. Epidemiology: The foundation of public health. In: Detels R, Gulliford M, Karim QA, Tan CC, eds. *Oxford Textbook of Global Public Health*. 6th ed. Oxford: Oxford University Press; 2015.
20. Kabir R, Khan H. Utilization of antenatal care among pregnant women of urban slums of Dhaka City, Bangladesh. *IOSR J Nurs Health Sci*. 2013;2(2):8–14.
21. Merrill RM. *Introduction to Epidemiology*. 7th ed. Burlington: Jones & Bartlett Learning; 2015.
22. Snow J. On the mode of communication of cholera. *Edinb Med J*. 1856;1(7):668–70.

2

Transmission of Communicable Diseases and Concepts of Disease Causation

Russell Kabir

The primary objective of public health is the prevention of diseases. To design prevention programs for diseases, it is vital to have a clear understanding of the causes of disease occurrence and the ways in which communicable diseases are transmitted. In this chapter, transmission of communicable diseases and the modern concepts of disease causation, pertinent to both communicable and noncommunicable diseases, are discussed.

2.1 Transmission of Communicable Diseases

Communicable diseases, also known as infectious diseases, are illnesses caused by pathogens (like bacteria, viruses, fungi, or parasites) that can be transmitted from one person to another. Communicable diseases constitute the major proportion of disease burden and are the leading cause of morbidity and mortality in the least developed countries. In 2019, 13.7 million people worldwide died from infectious syndromes, and three million of these deaths occurred in children under the age of five years. Globally, respiratory infections and bloodstream infections are the deadliest [1]. Poor people, women, children, the undernourished, and the elderly are the most vulnerable. Socioeconomic, environmental, and behavioral factors, as well as international travel and migration, foster and increase the spread of communicable diseases.

Communicable diseases refer to the diseases that are caused by an infectious agent that can be transmitted to other people from an infected person, animal, or a source in the environment. They are caused by certain types of infectious agents (pathogens), such as bacteria, viruses, parasites, and fungi, which invade the body and multiply or release toxins to cause damage to normal body cells and their functions. Understanding the different ways of transmission of a communicable disease is important to break the transmission chain and prevent the spread of the disease in the community. In low-income countries and among marginalized communities, communicable diseases like HIV/AIDS, tuberculosis (TB), malaria, viral hepatitis, and neglected tropical diseases (NTDs) are among the leading causes of mortality and disability. Having already taken the lives of 36.3 million people, HIV remains a serious global public health concern. TB is the second-most lethal infectious disease in the world, killing 1.5 million people a year. Seventy-seven percent (487,000) of all malaria deaths globally in 2020 occurred in children under five. Over one billion people received treatment for at least one of the five NTDs that can be prevented, controlled, or eliminated in the same year [2].

2.1.1 Transmission Cycle

Microorganisms live everywhere in our environment. People normally carry them on their skin, upper respiratory, intestinal, and genital tracts. In addition, microorganisms also live in animals, plants, soil, water, and air. Some organisms have more potential to cause disease.

The traditional epidemiologic triad model says that infectious diseases result from the interaction of *agent, host, and environment*. More specifically, transmission occurs when an infectious agent leaves its reservoir (host) through a portal of exit, conveyed by some mode of transmission, and enters through an appropriate portal of entry to infect a susceptible host. This sequence is sometimes called the transmission cycle or chain. The factors associated with the transmission cycle include: a) Infectious agent; b) Reservoir; c) Route of exit; d) Mode of transmission; e) Route of entry; and f) Susceptible host [3]

2.1.2 Infectious Agents

The microorganisms (infectious agents) that cause infections are known as pathogens. An infectious agent may be a bacterium, virus, protozoan, helminth, or fungus. Infectious agents can survive both in living subjects and non-living objects. Some agents can only persist and multiply inside human beings (e.g., HIV), whereas others can survive in animals (e.g., rabies and Japanese B encephalitis) or in the environment, such as soil or water (e.g., hookworm, cholera, and hepatitis A). The microorganisms may be classified as follows:

> *Bacteria:* Bacteria (e.g., Vibrio cholerae, Salmonella typhi, Shigella) are minute organisms approximately one-thousandth to five-thousandths of a millimeter in diameter. They are susceptible to a greater or lesser

extent to antibiotics. It is estimated that bacteria constitute approximately 38% of human pathogens.

Viruses: Viruses (e.g., HIV, hepatitis, and coronavirus) are much smaller than bacteria. Although they may survive outside the body for a short period of time, they can only grow inside the cells. Viruses are not susceptible to conventional antibiotics. There are a few anti-viral drugs available which are active against a limited number of viruses. About 44% of the diseases considered emerging in humans are viral.

Fungi: Fungi can be either moulds or yeasts. For example, a mould which causes infections in humans is *Trichophyton rubrum* (also called ringworm), which may infect the skin and nails. A common yeast infection is thrush, caused by *Candida albicans.*

Protozoa: Protozoa are microscopic organisms, but larger than bacteria. The pathogenic protozoa that commonly infect human beings are *Entamoeba histolytica* (causing diarrhea), *Giardia lamblia* (causing diarrhea), *and Plasmodium vivax* (causing malaria).

Worms: Worms are not always microscopic in size, but pathogenic worms do cause infection, and some can spread from person to person. Examples include threadworm, roundworm, and tapeworm.

Prions: Prions are infectious protein particles. All known prion diseases affect the structure of the brain or other neural tissue, and all are currently untreatable and universally fatal. Example: A prion is responsible for Creutzfeldt-Jakob disease.

2.1.3 Reservoir

The reservoir of an infectious agent is the habitat in which the agent normally lives, grows, and multiplies. Without reservoirs, infectious agents cannot survive and cannot be transmitted to other people. Humans and animals that serve as reservoirs are known as *infected hosts.* The reservoir may or may not be the source from which an agent is directly transferred to a host. For example, the reservoir of Japanese B encephalitis virus (JEV) is pigs, but the virus is transmitted through mosquitoes. Reservoirs include humans, animals, and the environment. When non-living things, like water, food, or soil, are the reservoirs for infectious agents, they are called *vehicles* (not infected hosts).

Human reservoirs: For many infectious diseases, humans are the reservoirs, and the diseases are transmitted from person to person without any mediator. These include sexually transmitted diseases (like gonorrhea, HIV, and syphilis), measles, mumps, streptococcal infection, and many respiratory pathogens. Human reservoirs may or may not have clinical manifestations. A carrier is a person with an inapparent infection (without having any symptoms or appearing healthy) and can transmit the disease to others.

Animal reservoirs: Many infectious agents are transmitted from animals to humans as incidental hosts. The term *zoonosis* refers to an infectious disease that is transmitted from vertebrate animals to humans. Some of the important zoonotic diseases include plague (from rodents), anthrax (from sheep), brucellosis (from cows and pigs), and rabies (from dogs or other wild animals).

Environmental reservoirs: Plants, soil, and water in the environment are also the reservoirs for some infectious agents. Many fungal agents, such as histoplasmosis, live and multiply in the soil. Hookworm is another example that is transmitted through contaminated soil.

2.1.4 Routes of Exit

Before an infectious agent can be transmitted to other people, it must first get out of the infected host. The site through which the infectious agent gets out of the infected host is called the route or portal of exit. The portal of exit usually corresponds to the site where the pathogen is localized. The common routes of exit are described below.

Respiratory tract: The routes of exit from the respiratory tract are the nose and mouth. Some infectious agents get out of the infected host in droplets expelled during coughing, sneezing, talking or spitting, and then get transmitted to others. For example, the agents for tuberculosis, COVID-19, measles, mumps, and influenza exit through the respiratory tract.

Gastrointestinal tract: The anus is the route of exit from the gastrointestinal tract. Some infectious agents, such as cholera, shigella, and hepatitis A, leave the human body through the faeces, and people are infected through contamination of food, water, or unclean hands.

Genitourinary tract: Infectious agents like HIV, syphilis, and gonorrhoea exit through the genitourinary tract, while Schistosomes exit through the urine.

Skin: Some infectious agents can exit the body through breaches in the skin. For example, this route of exit is used by Plasmodium protozoa (malarial parasites), which are present in the blood and get out of the human body when a mosquito bites through the skin to suck blood. Other examples are HIV and hepatitis B infections through cuts or needle stick injuries.

Placenta: Some blood-borne disease agents, such as rubella, syphilis, and HIV, can exit by crossing the placenta from mother to fetus.

2.1.5 Modes of Transmission

Once an infectious agent leaves a reservoir, it must be transmitted to a susceptible host to cause disease. The route by which an infectious agent is transmitted from a reservoir to another host is called the mode of transmission. The infectious diseases are transmitted from person to person by direct or indirect contact. How the disease is transmitted from one person to another depends on the type of disease or infectious agent. The following are the common ways of transmission of communicable diseases.

2.1.5.1 Direct Transmission

Direct transmission refers to the transfer of an infectious agent from an infected person to a new host without the need for intermediates, such as food, water, or insects. Direct modes of transmission can occur in two main ways. Diseases that can be transmitted by direct contact are called *contagious* diseases.

Person-to-person transmission: The infectious agent is spread by direct contact between people through touching, kissing, biting, or sexual intercourse (e.g., HIV, scabies, and fungal infections). Direct projection of respiratory droplets into another person's nose or mouth during coughing, sneezing, or talking is also considered direct transmission (such as COVID-19, pertussis, and meningococcal infection). Droplet transmission requires people to be near each other, approximately one meter (three feet) apart.

Transplacental transmission: This refers to the transmission of an infectious agent from a pregnant woman to her fetus through the placenta. An example is mother-to-child transmission of HIV [4].

2.1.5.2 Indirect Transmission

Indirect transmission is when infectious agents are transmitted to new hosts through some intermediates, such as air, food, water, animals, or objects in the environment. The following are the indirect modes of transmission.

Airborne transmission: Airborne transmission occurs when infectious agents are carried by dust or droplet nuclei from the respiratory tract suspended in air. Droplet nuclei are dried particles of less than five microns (μm) in size. In contrast to droplets that fall to the ground within a few feet, droplet nuclei may remain suspended in the air for long periods of time and may spread over greater distances. For example, measles, tuberculosis, and chicken pox can enter a new host through airborne transmission.

Vehicle-borne transmission: A vehicle is a non-living substance or object that can become contaminated by an infectious agent, which then transmits the disease to a new host. Examples of vehicles include water (which can spread cholera, dysentery, and hepatitis A), biological products (such as blood or serum, which may transmit HIV and hepatitis B), and food (which can spread typhoid, shigellosis, and hepatitis A).

Vector-borne transmission: Vectors are living invertebrate animals, such as mosquitoes, fleas, ticks, and houseflies. The vectors may transmit a disease mechanically (mechanical transmission) or may support the growth or changes of the agent (biological transmission). Examples of mechanical transmission are flies that carry shigella or vibrios (cholera organisms), and fleas that carry the causative agent of plague (*Yersinia pestis*) in their gut. On the other hand, in biological transmission, the causative agent undergoes maturation in an intermediate host before it can be transmitted to humans, e.g., mosquitoes transmit malaria, dengue, and yellow fever [4].

2.1.6 Routes of Entry

The site through which an infectious agent enters the host is called the route or portal of entry. The portal of entry must provide access to tissues where the pathogen can multiply. Often, infectious agents use the same portal of entry and exit of a host. For example, the influenza virus exits the respiratory tract of the source and enters the respiratory tract of the new host. On the other hand, many pathogens causing gastroenteritis follow the "fecal-oral" route because the organism exists through feces and enters the new host (either through unclean hands, contaminated food, or water) through the mouth (e.g., shigellosis and cholera). Other portals of entry include the skin (hookworm), mucous membranes (syphilis), placenta (HIV), urinary tract (gonorrhea), and blood (hepatitis B and HIV) [5].

2.1.7 Susceptible Host

After an infectious agent gets inside the body, it must multiply in order to cause the disease. In some hosts, infection leads to the disease, but in others it does not. Individuals who are likely to develop a communicable disease after exposure to infectious agents are called susceptible hosts.

Not all individuals are equally susceptible to infection for various reasons. Susceptibility of a host depends on genetic or other factors, such as immunity and nonspecific factors like general health and nutritional status that affect an individual's ability to resist infection. For example, persons with sickle cell disease are partially resistant to a particular type of malaria.

Immunity refers to the resistance of an individual to communicable diseases, which is due to the presence of protective antibodies against a specific agent. Such antibodies may be developed in response to an infection, a vaccine, or acquired through other means, such as transfer from mother to fetus or the injection of antibodies (e.g., tetanus antitoxin). Nonspecific factors that protect against infection include the skin, mucous membranes, gastric acidity, cough reflex, and nonspecific immune response.

Factors that increase the susceptibility of a host to the development of a communicable disease are called *risk factors*. Some risk factors arise from outside the individual – for example, poor personal hygiene or poor control of reservoirs in the environment. Such factors increase the exposure of the susceptible hosts to infectious agents, which makes the disease more likely to develop.

Additionally, some people in a community are more likely to develop the disease than others, even though they all have the same exposure to infectious agents. This is due to a low level of *immunity*. Low levels of immunity could be due to: a) Presence of other diseases, such as HIV and cancer, which suppress the body's immune system; b) Poorly developed or immature immunity, as in very young children or very old people; c) Not being vaccinated; d) Poor nutrition; and e) Pregnancy.

2.2 Iceberg of Disease

The term "iceberg of disease" is often used in epidemiology to describe the concept that visible and clinically diagnosed cases of a particular disease represent only a small portion of the total burden of that disease within a population.

Just like an iceberg, where most of its mass lies underwater and is hidden from view, a significant portion of the disease burden remains undetected or unnoticed (as shown in Figure 2.1).

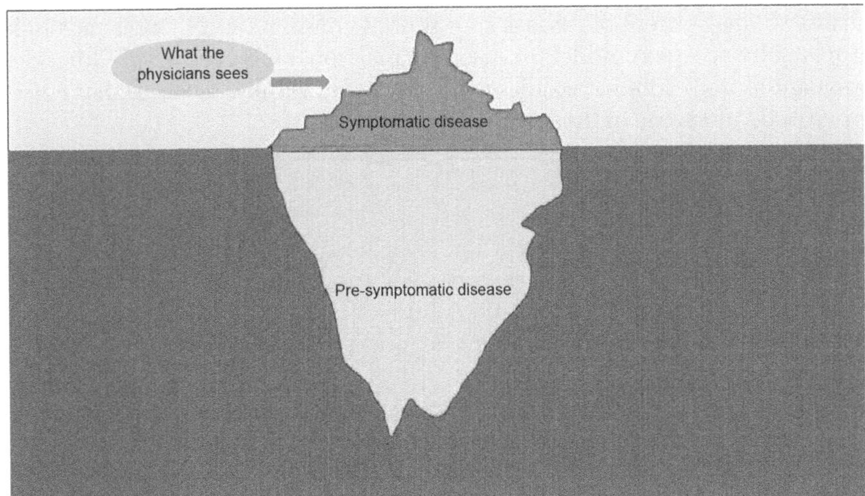

FIGURE 2.1
Iceberg of disease.

The iceberg of disease concept suggests that there are many asymptomatic or mildly symptomatic cases that go unreported and untreated. Because people do not seek medical assistance or because the symptoms are not severe enough to warrant medical attention, these situations may not be brought to the attention of public health authorities.

Only a small portion of the population's actual problems are visible or diagnosed, which is the tip of the iceberg. In addition to confirmed cases, the true burden of the disease also includes undiagnosed and subclinical cases that are not counted in official statistics. Understanding the iceberg of disease is crucial for public health officials and policymakers because it highlights the importance of surveillance, early detection, and prevention efforts. By recognizing that there are many unreported cases, public health measures can be implemented to stop the disease's spread, lessen its effects, and ultimately safeguard the population's health. This idea is especially pertinent when it comes to infectious diseases because early detection and intervention can help stop outbreaks and lessen the overall strain on healthcare systems [6].

2.3 Concepts of Disease Causation

The concept of disease causation is an essential component of epidemiological science that explores the factors or agents responsible for the occurrence of a disease. This concept involves investigating the underlying factors responsible for the onset of a disease in the population, and understanding the causes of disease is crucial in the prevention, diagnosis, and treatment of diseases. The concept of disease causation is complex, and there is no single, universally accepted model for disease causation. However, several theories, relevant to both communicable and non-communicable diseases, have been proposed, and some of them are discussed here.

2.3.1 Epidemiologic Triad

In epidemiology, a few models for the causation of a disease have been proposed. Among them, the *epidemiologic triad* is the traditional and commonly used model for the causation of infectious diseases. The triad consists of an external agent, a susceptible host, and an environment that brings the host and agent together.

According to the epidemiological triad model, transmission occurs when the agent leaves the reservoir or host through a portal of exit, and is conveyed by a mode of transmission to enter through an appropriate portal of entry to infect the susceptible host. Transmission may be direct or indirect. This concept states that for a disease to occur, there must be a unique combination of events, that is, a harmful agent that comes into contact with a susceptible host in a proper environment.

Here is an example of an epidemiological triad for the disease measles:

- Agent: Measles virus.
- Host: Susceptible individual or population.
- Environment: Close contact with an infected person.

When all three components of the epidemiological triad are present, measles can occur. The measles virus is highly contagious and spreads through respiratory droplets produced when an infected person coughs or sneezes.

2.3.2 Web of Causation

The web of causation model depicts that three categories of factors are interconnected and can influence each other in a bidirectional manner. For example, a genetic predisposition to disease may interact with environmental factors, such as exposure to certain pollutants or lifestyle choices, to determine whether an individual develops the disease. Similarly, social and cultural factors may influence behaviors (e.g., smoking or eating habits), which, in turn, can impact health outcomes. The model also recognizes that disease causation is often a result of multiple causative factors working together rather than a single cause. This understanding highlights the importance of considering the broader context and interactions between various factors when addressing public health issues.

2.3.3 Multifactorial Causation

According to multifactorial causation of disease, apart from the causal agent, there are many other factors responsible for the causation of the disease, such as social, economic, cultural, genetic, and psychological. For example, while tubercle bacilli are the primary cause of tuberculosis, factors such as poverty, overcrowding, malnutrition, and genetic predispositions also play an important role in its occurrence.

2.3.4 Causal Pie

The causal pie model is a conceptual framework used in the field of epidemiology to understand the causes of diseases or health outcomes. It helps to identify and quantify various factors that contribute to the development of a particular condition. The model suggests that an outcome, such as a disease, is the result of multiple causal factors that act independently or interact with each other. In the causal pie model, the total causal effect is represented by a pie, and each causal factor is depicted as a slice of the pie. The size of each slice represents the magnitude of the effect that factor has on the outcome. The sum of all the slices in the pie equals the total causal effect. The model emphasizes that no single factor is solely responsible for the outcome. Instead, multiple factors, including genetic predisposition, environmental exposures, lifestyle choices, and social determinants, contribute to the development of a disease. The model assumes that causal factors act independently and additively, which may not always be the case. Additionally, there may be interactions and feedback loops between different factors that influence the outcome. Despite these limitations, the causal pie model provides a valuable framework for understanding the multifactorial nature of disease causation and guiding public health interventions. For example, smoking is a well-known risk factor for lung cancer. Other factors that may contribute to lung cancer include exposure to environmental pollutants, genetic predisposition, occupational hazards (such as exposure to asbestos), and lifestyle factors like diet and physical activity.

2.3.5 Sufficient-Component Cause Model

Sufficient-component cause models are another conceptual framework used in epidemiology to understand the causes of diseases or health outcomes. The models focus on identifying the necessary and sufficient conditions that lead to the development of a particular outcome. In a sufficient-component cause model, a disease or outcome is seen as the result of a combination of multiple factors, each of which is necessary but not sufficient on its own. These factors can be biological, environmental, behavioral, or social in nature. When all the necessary components come together, they form a sufficient cause that leads to the outcome.

This model emphasizes that different pathways can lead to the same outcome and that multiple combinations of factors can result in the development of a disease. It also recognizes that the absence of a particular factor can prevent the outcome from occurring, even if other factors are present. Sufficient-component cause models are useful in understanding the complexity of disease causation and identifying potential intervention points for prevention and control. However, like the causal pie model, they have limitations in capturing the full complexity of real-world causality. For example, HIV exposure is necessary for AIDS to occur, and TB exposure is necessary for TB infection to occur.

2.4 Commonly Used Definitions in Epidemiology

Attack rate
This is similar to the cumulative incidence, but it does not have the time factor. This term is commonly used in foodborne outbreaks, where the outbreak

occurs within a few hours or days. In a broad sense, it is a proportion rather than a rate. It is calculated as the number of people who ate a certain food and got sick (numerator) divided by the total number of people who ate the same food (denominator).

Secondary attack rate
First, we have to understand what a primary case and a secondary case are. A primary case is the person who developed the disease after exposure (e.g., contaminated food). Secondary case is the case (person) who developed the disease after coming into contact with the primary case. The secondary attack rate is therefore defined as the attack rate among the suspected people who were exposed to the primary case. It is calculated as: the number of people who developed the disease after exposure to the primary case (numerator) divided by the total number of people who were exposed to the primary case (denominator).

Epidemic
An epidemic is defined as the occurrence of a group of illnesses of a similar nature clearly in *excess of normal expectancy,* in a community or region. The occurrence of a single case of a communicable disease that was absent for a long time in a population, or the occurrence of a single case for the first time (not previously recognized) in the community, is also considered an epidemic. An epidemic can be of:

- Point source epidemic (or common source epidemic)
  Here, an epidemic/outbreak occurs from a standard vehicle such as food, salad, or water. In a common source outbreak, many people are exposed to the etiologic agent simultaneously. The cases occur rapidly after the first onset, reach a peak, and then decline. The duration of the epidemic is within the range of the incubation period.

- Propagated epidemic
  Here, the disease is transmitted from human or animal reservoirs by direct or indirect contact with a host. For a propagated epidemic, a large majority of the population is non-immune (susceptible to infection). Periodic contact with the infected person is essential for the continuous spread of the disease.

Endemic
It is defined as the *habitual presence* of a disease within a given geographical area. It may also refer to the usual occurrence of a given disease within the area, e.g., malaria is endemic in many parts of the world. Endemic can be:

- Hyper endemic
  It means the disease is constantly present at a high incidence or prevalence rate and affects all age groups equally, e.g., dengue fever.

- Holo endemic
  This kind of endemic disease affects most individuals in a population and the infection is highly prevalent in the early years of life, e.g., malaria.

Pandemic
When an epidemic affects several countries simultaneously worldwide, diseases that have the potential to cause a pandemic include COVID-19, plague, and cholera.

Sporadic
Occurrence of a small number of cases of disease here and there, e.g., polio-myelitis and chicken pox.

Exotic
Diseases that do not occur in a country under normal conditions but are imported from another country, e.g., yellow fever in Bangladesh.

Epizootic
When there is an outbreak of disease in the animal population, there is an implication that it may also transfer to the human population. Only a few zoonotic agents can cause such outbreaks, e.g., anthrax, brucellosis, rabies, influenza, Rift Valley fever, Q fever, and Japanese encephalitis.

Control
Control means cessation of disease progress in a specific population group of an area or region from which it is not a threat to public health anymore, e.g., TB, Polio, leprosy, and Malaria.

Eradication
The complete extinction of disease and the permanent stamping out of its causes is called the eradication of disease. For example, smallpox has been eradicated from the globe.

Elimination
The term elimination is used when it is not possible to completely eradicate a disease, i.e., elimination of neonatal tetanus is defined as bringing the incidence less than one per 1,000 live births per year.

Isolation
Isolation separates sick people with a contagious disease from people who are not ill. For example, if you have tested positive for COVID-19, though you are not showing any symptoms.

Quarantine
Quarantine separates and restricts the movement of people who were exposed to a contagious disease to see if they become sick. For example, when a person stays away from others after being in close contact with someone who is COVID-19 positive.

Herd Immunity
Herd immunity occurs when a large proportion of a population becomes immune to an infectious disease, reducing the risk of spread from one person to another, and those who are not immune are indirectly protected because ongoing disease spread is minimal. Vaccination is the best way to develop herd immunity in the community.

Virulence
This is the ability of an organism to infect the host and cause disease, e.g., Botulinum toxin, produced by Clostridium botulinum, causes botulism, a severe food poisoning illness.

Infectivity
This is the ability of an infectious agent to invade and multiply, thus producing infection in a host.

Opportunistic infection
An infection that takes advantage of the weak immune system of the body to infect the host is called an opportunistic infection. Organisms such as Herpes simplex, Cytomegalovirus, and Toxoplasma are generally not pathogenic but can cause disease when the immune system weakens.

Nosocomial infection
It is also known as a hospital-acquired infection or healthcare-associated infection. Generally, when patients develop any infection originating from the hospital setting, it is called a nosocomial infection. It develops a new disorder, different from the patient's primary condition, associated with being in the hospital. Generally, the infection is acquired in the hospital or develops after discharge, e.g., surgical wound infection, catheter-induced urinary tract infection, and pneumonia.

Iatrogenic infection
It is a clinical condition that results from the direct or indirect actions of health care professionals. Iatrogenic diseases include anything that is caused by a diagnostic procedure or treatment, such as medication, radiation, or surgery. For example, a pneumothorax develops because of thoracentesis.

Contamination
The presence of an infectious agent on body surfaces, clothes, beds, surgical equipment, or other inanimate objects or substances, including water, milk, and food. For example, microbial agents are responsible for food contamination, which can be transferred from a farm.

Community transmission
The term community transmission means that the source of infection for the spread of an illness is unknown, i.e., a link in terms of contact between patients and other people is missing.

Prevention
Measures taken before the occurrence of a communicable disease to protect
an individual or community from getting it, and to reduce the number of
cases locally in the future. For example, vaccination, improved nutrition,
hand washing, and the use of insecticide-treated mosquito nets (ITNs) to prevent malaria.

Pathogenicity
This is the ability of an infectious agent to induce clinically apparent illness.
For example, pathogenic agents are infectious bacteria, viruses, fungi, and
parasites causing disease.

References

1.   Gray A, Sharara F. Global and regional sepsis and infectious syndrome mor-
      tality in 2019: A systematic analysis. *Lancet Glob Health.* 2022;10:S2.
2.   World Health Organization. *Communicable and Noncommunicable Diseases
      and Mental Health.* Available from: www.who.int/our-work/communicable-
      and-noncommunicable-diseases-and-mental-health
3.   OpenLearnCreate. *Basic Concepts in the Transmission of Communicable Diseases.*
      Available from: www.open.edu/openlearncreate/mod/oucontent/view.
      php?id=84&printable=1
4.   OpenLearnCreate. *Basic Concepts of the Transmission of Communicable
      Diseases: The Natural History of a Disease.* Available from: www.open.edu/
      openlearncreate/mod/oucontent/view.php?id=84&printable=1#:~:text=
      The%20natural%20history%20of%20an,disease%2C%20and%20stage%20
      of%20outcome
5.   Centers for Disease Control and Prevention. *Principles of Epidemiology in
      Public Health Practice: An Introduction to Applied Epidemiology and Biostatistics.*
      3rd ed. Available from: /www.cdc.gov/csels/dsepd/ss1978/lesson1/sectio
      n10.html
6.   Centers for Disease Control and Prevention. *Quarantine and Isolation.* 2017.
      Available from: www.cdc.gov/quarantine/index.html

3

Measures of Morbidity and Mortality

Mohammad Tajul Islam

Epidemiology is primarily a quantitative method. In Chapter 1, we discussed that the objectives of epidemiology are to describe the distribution and identify the determinants of disease in the community. Therefore, epidemiology encompasses both the description of the disease patterns in terms of its occurrence in the human population and the identification of factors associated with disease. To achieve these objectives, it is essential to measure the frequency of disease or other outcomes of interest. Such information serves as the basic tool for the comparison of disease frequencies among different populations for the formulation and testing of hypotheses.

In general, methods used for describing the disease patterns are the measures of mortality and morbidity. The first one (mortality) provides data on the occurrence of deaths, while the latter (morbidity) provides data on the occurrence of sickness. The measurement of morbidity data is more complex than that of mortality data. While measuring morbidities, there may be more subclinical cases (which cannot be detected) than the number of sick individuals, and an individual may suffer from a number of episodes of an illness in a given time period. Moreover, a person may have several illnesses during a given time interval. All these factors make the morbidity data more complex to handle. In this chapter, the basic measurements of morbidity and mortality and how they are calculated are discussed.

3.1 Basic Tools of Epidemiology: Count, Rate, Ratio, and Proportion

3.1.1 Count

Counting the occurrence of a disease is a very basic measurement. Such information helps the health manager decide about intervention and allocation of resources. However, disease patterns in terms of mortality and morbidity cannot be described by numbers alone, and the count data have very limited utility in epidemiology [1, 2].

The other pieces of information necessary for the measurement of morbidity and mortality include the population size from which the numbers were derived and the time period during which data were collected. Such information allows us to compare the disease frequencies in two or more groups of individuals (i.e., populations).

Table 3.1 shows the hypothetical data on the frequency of malaria in two districts for the year 2020. Looking at the number of malaria cases reported from the districts, one may falsely conclude that malaria is more common in District A than in District B (since the number of reported cases is higher in District A). To make the data comparable, we need to consider the population size from which the cases are derived and the time period during which the numbers have been reported. In this example, we can see that the rate of malaria in District B is 158.3 per 100,000 population per year, which is higher than that of District A.

Therefore, instead of counting alone, other measures of morbidity and mortality, such as rate, ratio, and proportion, are used as the basic tools in epidemiology for better description of disease patterns and comparison [1–9].

3.1.2 Rate

Rate is a special form of proportion that includes a specification of time. In epidemiology, rate is a measure of the frequency of a disease (or an event) that occurs in a defined population over a specified time period. Rate is a very basic measurement since it expresses the probability or risk of the occurrence of a disease in a population. It has a numerator, a denominator, and a multiplier (constant). Here, the numerator is included in the denominator. The rate has a time period, while the proportion is not time-bound. Rate is commonly expressed as a percentage, per 1,000, per 100,000, or others. Examples of rates are the incidence rate, crude birth rate, neonatal mortality rate, and attack rate. The properties and uses of rate are:

TABLE 3.1

Number of reported cases of malaria in two districts (hypothetical data)

Location	No. of cases	Period	Total population
District A	270	January to December 2020	220,000
District B	190	January to December 2020	120,000

Annual rate of occurrence of malaria:
District A: (270 ÷ 220,000) × 100,000 = 122.7 per 100,000 population per year
District B: (190 ÷ 120,000) × 100,000 = 158.3 per 100,000 population per year

- Rate is a commonly used measure of morbidity and mortality in epidemiology. It is used mainly as a descriptive tool. For example, the incidence rate of a disease, the crude death rate, and the neonatal mortality rate.
- Rate is always time-bound (i.e., reported per unit of time).
- Rate is particularly useful for comparing disease frequency in different populations, geographical locations, and at different times.

A rate can be calculated as:

$$\frac{\text{No. of events}\left(\text{e.g., a disease}\right)\text{in a specified period}}{\text{No. of population at risk of the event in the same specified period}} \times K\left(\text{constant}\right)$$

Example

In a district with a population of 2,000,000, there were 14,050 deaths in the year 2019. The crude death rate (CDR) for the district in 2019 is, therefore, $(14{,}050 \div 2{,}000{,}000) \times 1{,}000 = 7.03$ per 1,000 population.

3.1.3 Ratio

A ratio expresses the relationship between two numbers in the form of X:Y or $(X \div Y)$. In other words, a ratio indicates the relative magnitude of two quantities or a comparison of two values. It is the expression of the relationship between a numerator and a denominator. The numerator and denominator need not be related. In a ratio, the numerator is usually not included in the denominator. The constant (multiplier) is usually one or 100. For example, the doctor-patient ratio at a hospital is one to ten (i.e., for every ten patients, there is one doctor).

In certain ratios, the numerator and denominator are different categories of the same variable (e.g., gender), such as the ratio of males to females (e.g., the ratio of male and female patients attending the emergency department of a hospital). In other ratios, the numerator and denominator are completely different variables, such as the number of nurses and the number of doctors in a hospital (e.g., nurse-to-doctor ratio). The properties and uses of ratio are:

- Ratios can be used as both descriptive and analytic tools. Examples of descriptive measures are the male-to-female ratio of patients attending the emergency department, the case-to-control ratio of a case-control study, and the doctor-to-nurse ratio at a hospital. As an analytic measure, a ratio is used to calculate the risk of occurrence of a disease, such as the risk ratio (also called relative risk), odds ratio, and rate ratio.
- Usually, the values of both the numerator and denominator of a ratio are divided by the value of one or the other so that either the numerator or the

denominator equals one. For example, in a hospital, there are 250 male and 100 female staff. Therefore, the ratio of male-to-female staff is 2.5:1.

3.1.4 Proportion

A proportion is the comparison of a part to the whole. It is a type of ratio where the numerator is always included in the denominator and is usually expressed as a percentage (multiplier is 100). The proportion does not have a time factor. For example, the proportion of women who had home deliveries, the proportion of health facilities that provide emergency obstetric care services, and the proportion of males of all COVID-19 patients admitted to a hospital. The properties and uses of proportion are:

- Proportions are common descriptive measures used in epidemiology. For example, the proportion of deliveries conducted at health facilities and the proportion of children under one immunized against measles.

- Proportions are also used to describe the amount of disease that can be attributed to a particular exposure. For example, 40% of tuberculosis cases are attributed to malnutrition.

- In a proportion, the numerator is always included in the denominator.

- A proportion can also be expressed as a fraction, a decimal, or a percentage.

Example
A study was conducted in a district, taking a random sample of 600 women who had a delivery within one year prior to the data collection. The study showed that out of 600 women, 259 had their deliveries at health facilities. Therefore, the proportion of women who delivered at health facilities in the district is $(259 \div 600) \times 100 = 43.2\%$.

3.2 Measures of Morbidity and Mortality: Prevalence and Incidence

3.2.1 Prevalence

Prevalence is a commonly used measure of morbidity in epidemiology. Prevalence is the existing number of cases of a disease (or other condition) in a given population at a certain point in time (point prevalence) or over a period of time (period prevalence). In literature, the term "prevalence rate" is frequently used interchangeably with "prevalence". By definition, prevalence is not a rate but a proportion.

Prevalence is an important measure in epidemiology, especially for chronic diseases, such as diabetes, hypertension, and asthma. The prevalence data help the health managers to understand the disease burden in the community and plan for intervention. Prevalence data also help in monitoring intervention programs. Periodical estimation of point prevalence is useful in tracking changes in disease patterns over time. Prevalence data sometimes also suggest the possible etiology of a disease [1–3]. There are two types of measures of prevalence: a) point prevalence and b) period prevalence.

3.2.1.1 Point Prevalence

Point prevalence is the frequency of a disease in a certain population at a certain point in time. It indicates the proportion of persons with a particular disease in a population on a particular date. Point prevalence is the measure of estimated prevalence in a cross-sectional study or survey. For example, the prevalence of hypertension among adults (18 to 69 years) in Bangladesh is 21.0% [10]. Point prevalence is calculated as:

$$\text{Point prevalence} = \frac{\begin{array}{c}\text{No. of existing cases of a disease in} \\ \text{the population at a specified time}\end{array}}{\begin{array}{c}\text{No. of persons in the population} \\ \text{(or surveyed) at that specified time}\end{array}} \times K$$

Here, K is the multiplier (constant) that can be 100, 1,000, 100,000, or others.

Example
A survey was conducted in December 2019, taking a random sample from a district. The study showed that out of 700 children under the age of five, 98 were undernourished. Therefore, the point prevalence of undernutrition among the under-five children in the district is 14.0% (98 ÷ 700 × 100). Other examples are the findings of the Bangladesh Demographic and Health Surveys (BDHS), such as the contraceptive prevalence rate, prevalence of diabetes, and prevalence of hypertension.

Point prevalence is a useful index to express the magnitude of a current health problem and is important to health managers and policy makers. Point prevalence is the basis for calculating the prevalence ratio, a measure of association in cross-sectional studies. In a situation where incidence and duration of the disease are stable and in-migration equals out-migration, the relationship between prevalence and incidence can be expressed as:

$$\text{Point prevalence} = \text{Incidence} \times \text{Average duration of the disease}$$

3.2.1.2 Period Prevalence

Period prevalence is less commonly used. It is defined as the number of cases of a disease in a population during a defined period of time. For instance, for the calculation of the period prevalence of a disease in 2020, the numerator is the number of existing cases of the disease on 1 January 2020, plus all the new cases (incidence cases) that occurred during the year (from 2 January to 31 December 2020). In period prevalence, the denominator is the average reference population (*mid-year population*) of the defined period in the area.

$$\text{Period prevalence} = \frac{\text{No. of cases of a disease (old \& new) at specified time interval}}{\text{Mid}-\text{year population in the area druing the defined period}} \times K$$

Here, K is the multiplier (constant) that can be 100, 1,000, 100,000, or others.

Example
Assume that a village had 2,000 people on 1 January 2020, and 2,050 people on 31 December 2020. On 1 January there were 35 cases of asthma in the village, and five persons developed asthma (new cases) between 2 January and 31 December 2020. What is the period prevalence of asthma for the year 2020?

   To calculate the period prevalence, first calculate the mid-year population of the village. The mid-year population is the average of the population at the beginning (on 1 January; 2,000) and end (31 December; 2,050) of the specified period (2020). The mid-year population of the village (for 2020) is 2,025 [(2,000 + 2050) ÷ 2]. The period prevalence of asthma for the year 2020 is 1.98% [(35 + 5) ÷ 2025 × 100)]. From the data, we can also calculate the point prevalence on 1 January [(35 ÷ 2,000) × 100 = 1.75%] and on 31 December [(40 ÷ 2,050) × 100) = 1.95%].

3.2.2 Incidence

Incidence is measured in prospective (follow-up) studies. It measures the probability that a healthy person will develop a disease in a specified period of time (cumulative incidence) or how quickly the disease occurs in a population (incidence rate). Incidence is commonly defined as the number of new cases of a disease (or an event) in a defined population over a specified period of time (numerator) divided by the number of individuals at risk for the same disease (or event) during that time period (denominator). To calculate the incidence of a disease for a population, the following conditions need to be fulfilled [1–3]:

- The population must be free from the disease of interest at the beginning of the study;

- The population must be at risk of developing the disease; and
- The population must be followed for a certain period of time for the occurrence of new cases.

Depending on the type of denominator, there are two types of measures of incidence [3, 6]. They are:

- Incidence based on *persons at risk* (cumulative incidence); and
- Incidence based on *person-time units at risk* (incidence rate or incidence density).

3.2.2.1 Cumulative Incidence Based on Persons at Risk

The incidence of a disease where the denominator is the number of persons at risk is called *cumulative incidence or incidence proportion*. Cumulative incidence is basically a probability. It provides an estimate (probability) of the risk that a person will develop a disease during a specified time period. While reporting the cumulative incidence, the relevant time period must be clearly specified. Cumulative incidence is the basis for survival analysis.

While calculating the cumulative incidence from the data of a follow-up study, we may encounter two situations. First, a situation where all individuals were successfully followed until the end of the study period (i.e., there was no loss to follow-up), and second, a situation where all individuals could not be followed for the entire study period, i.e., there were losses to follow-up (attritions). Therefore, we need to consider these situations when calculating the cumulative incidence.

3.2.2.2 Cumulative Incidence When There Is No Loss to Follow-Up

In a follow-up study, if it is possible to follow all individuals up to the end of the study period without any attrition (lost to follow-up), the total number of individuals at the beginning of the study (population at risk) constitutes the denominator. The cumulative incidence (Cu. Ic.) is, therefore, the number of events (diseases or deaths) occurred during the specified time period (numerator) divided by the number of population at risk at the beginning of the study.

$$\text{Cu. Ic.} = \frac{\text{No. of new cases of a disease during a given time period}}{\text{No. of population at risk at the beginning of the study}} \times K$$

Here, K is the multiplier (constant) that can be 100, 1,000, 100,000, or others.

Example

A cohort study was conducted with 300 individuals with hypertension who were free from heart disease (myocardial infarction) at the beginning. They were followed for a period of two years. The objective was to estimate the cumulative incidence of heart disease (outcome of interest) among patients with hypertension. During the follow-up period, six individuals developed heart disease. Therefore, the two-year cumulative incidence of heart disease for that population is (6 ÷ 300) or 0.02 or 2.0% (or 1% per year).

As discussed before, the numerator for the calculation of incidence is the number of individuals who developed an event (disease, death, or others). In certain circumstances, an individual may suffer from several episodes of the same event in a specified time period, e.g., a number of episodes of diarrhea or the common cold. This gives rise to the calculation of two types of incidences from the same dataset. First, where the numerator is the *number of individuals* who developed the event (e.g., diarrhea) in one year, and second, the *number of episodes* of the event (e.g., diarrhea) that the individuals developed during a one-year period. The denominator in both these situations is the same, i.e., the total number of individuals at risk during the given time period. The incidence calculated with the first numerator indicates the probability (risk) of a person developing diarrhea (cumulative incidence), while the second numerator indicates the number of diarrheal episodes per person in a year (called incidence in spell).

Example

In a one-year follow-up study of 500 children under five years of age, it was observed that 200 children suffered from diarrhea at any time during the follow-up period. Of those who suffered from diarrhea, 40 children had diarrhea three times during the year. Thus, the total episodes of diarrhea among children were 280 [(40 × 3) + (160 × 1)].

Therefore, the cumulative incidence of diarrhea among children was 40% [(200 ÷ 500) × 100] per year, and the incidence in spells was 0.56 (280 ÷ 500) episodes per child per year or 56 episodes per 100 children per year.

3.2.2.3 Cumulative Incidence When There Are Losses to Follow-Up

In cohort studies, in most cases, follow-up of all individuals is not possible for the full length of the study period (complete follow-up), either because of losses to follow-up or because individuals are recruited later in the period for the study. Observations of individuals with incomplete follow-up are called *censored observations*.

Subjects may be lost to follow-up due to withdrawal, migration, or death due to other causes than the outcome of interest. Moreover, subjects may be recruited for the study at different points in the study period. All these factors cause a shorter duration of follow-up for some individuals. It, therefore, requires special attention during data analysis. Techniques that are used in such a situation (i.e., when there are attritions or censored observations) include the *Classic Life Table approach and the Kaplan-Meier approach* [3, 6].

3.2.2.4 Cumulative Incidence: Classic Life Table Approach

In the classic life table approach, the probability (incidence) of an event is not calculated for the entire follow-up period at a time. Instead, depending on the situation, the follow-up period is divided into several shorter time intervals, such as one-month, three-month, six-month, or one-year intervals, and the incidence is calculated separately for each interval. The denominator for the calculation of incidence is determined as:

$$\text{Denominator} = (\text{No. at the beginning}) - (\text{Half of individuals lost to follow} - \text{up})$$

Example

Suppose a researcher intends to determine the two-year incidence of death (the outcome of interest) following cardiac surgery. To conduct the study, ten patients who underwent cardiac surgery were recruited for a follow-up study. Figure 3.1 provides a schematic representation of the follow-up of these patients.

As shown in the figure, ten patients (labeled A to J) were recruited and followed for up to two years. Each horizontal line represents the follow-up

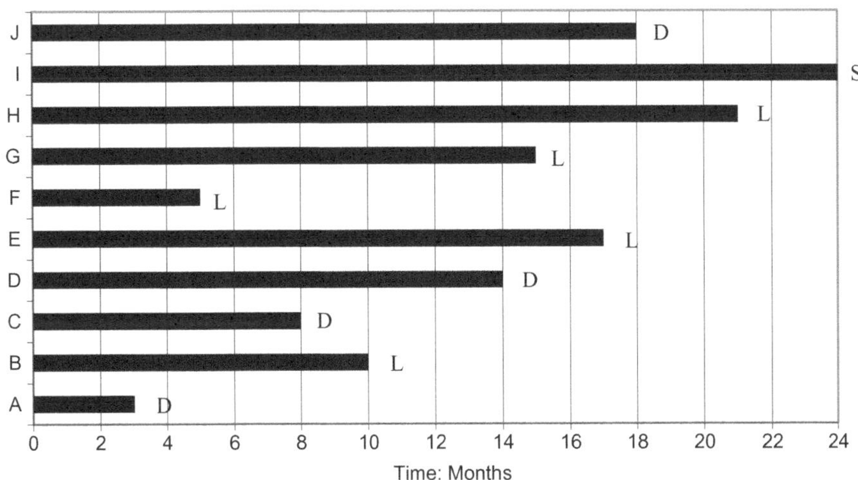

FIGURE 3.1
Follow-up of ten patients with cardiac surgery.

period for an individual. Of the recruited patients, four died (marked as "D"), and five were lost to follow-up (marked as "L") during the two-year study period. One patient was still alive at the end of the study period (marked as "S"). It is important to note that follow-up is terminated either by death (the event) or by loss to follow-up for any reason, as neither can contribute further to the study.

The life table calculates the incidence based on probability. In our example (Figure 3.1), there were four deaths during the follow-up period. If it were possible to follow all ten patients up to the end of the study without any attrition (loss), the cumulative incidence of death would have been (4 ÷ 10) or 0.40 or 40.0% for a period of two years.

However, since there are censored observations (subjects who were not followed for the entire two-year period or subjects who were not at risk for the entire two-year follow-up period), we need to consider this while calculating the incidence. To do this, half of the individuals who were lost to follow-up (i.e., 5 ÷ 2 = 2.5) will be subtracted from the denominator. Therefore, the denominator for the calculation of cumulative incidence will be 7.5 (10 − 2.5). The two-year cumulative incidence of death among patients with cardiac surgery is, therefore, 0.53 (4 ÷ 7.5), or 53.0%. Here, the assumption is that losses to follow-up occurred uniformly over the study period, thus giving the average population at risk. The complement of this measure (i.e., the incidence), 0.47 (1 − 0.53), is called the *survival probability* (in our example, 0.47 is the two-year survival probability).

In the classic life table approach, incidence is not calculated for the entire follow-up period at a time. The follow-up time is usually divided into multiple shorter time intervals to calculate the survival probabilities. For example, the two-year follow-up period may be divided into three-month, six-month, or one-year time intervals, and the survival probabilities are calculated at each time interval separately.

It is not necessary that the intervals in the life table approach be of the same duration. Intervals may vary depending on the situation, like changes in the risk of an event over time. For example, the risk of death after an acute heart attack is high during the initial one or two days, and the risk gradually decreases over time.

Let us consider the data provided in Figure 3.1 to calculate survival probabilities at every 6-month time interval, i.e., Interval 1 (0 to 6 months); Interval 2 (>6 to 12 months); Interval 3 (>12 to 18 months); and Interval 4 (>18 to 24 months). The incidences, survival probabilities, and cumulative survival probabilities are provided in Table 3.2 and are calculated using the classic life table approach.

Denominators (C4) are calculated as the number of people at risk at the beginning of the interval minus half the number of people lost to follow-up during that interval. Therefore, the denominators, in our example, are for (Table 3.2):

TABLE 3.2

Working table for the calculation of cumulative survival probability using the classic life table approach

Follow-up Interval in months	No. of people at risk	No. lost to follow-up	Actual no. at risk (Denominator)	No. of events during the interval (Numerator)	Incidence of event during the period	Probability of survival	Cumulative survival probability
C1	C2	C3	C4	C5	C6	C7	C8
0 to 6	10	1	9.5	1	0.105	0.895	0.895
>6 to 12	8	1	7.5	1	0.133	0.867	0.775
>12 to 18	6	2	5.0	2	0.400	0.600	0.465
>18 to 24	2	1	1.5	0	0.000	1.000	0.465

Calculations:

C4 (Denominator) $= C2 - (C3 \times 0.5)$

C6 (Incidence of event) $= (C5 \div C4)$

C7 (Survival probability) $= (1 - C6)$

C8 (Cumulative survival probability)
$= 0.896$ (same as C7) for 0 to 6 months interval
$= 0.896 \times 0.867$ for >6 to 12 months interval
$= 0.896 \times 0.867 \times 0.60$ for >12 to 18 months interval
$= 0.896 \times 0.867 \times 0.60 \times 1.0$ for >18 to 24 months interval

- Interval 1 (0 to 6 months) is $[10 - (1 \times 0.5)] = 9.5$;
- Interval 2 (>6 to 12 months) is 7.5 $[8 - (1 \times 0.5)]$ [no. of people at risk at the beginning of the interval is 8 (10 – no. lost to follow-up – no. of deaths in the previous interval)];
- Similarly, the denominators for intervals 3 (>12 to 18) and 4 (>18 to 24) are 5.0 and 1.5, respectively.

The incidence (or probability) of an event (C6) is calculated as $[C5 \div C4]$, while the survival probability (i.e., the probability of not having an event; C7) is calculated as $[1 - C6]$. The last column (C8) indicates the cumulative survival probabilities and is calculated as:

- Interval 1 (0 to 6 months): 0.895 [same as the survival probability].
- Interval 2 (>6 to 12 months): 0.895×0.867 [survival probability of Interval 1 × survival probability of Interval 2];
- Interval 3 (>12 to 18 months): $0.895 \times 0.867 \times 0.600$ [survival probability of Interval 1 × survival probability of Interval 2 × survival probability of Interval 3]; and
- Interval 4 (>18 to 24 months): $0.895 \times 0.867 \times 0.600 \times 1.0$ [survival probability of Interval 1 × survival probability of Interval 2 × survival probability of Interval 3 × survival probability of Interval 4].

Table 3.2 shows that the cumulative survival probability beyond two years is 0.465 or 46.5%. This means that the probability of surviving beyond two years among individuals after cardiac surgery is 46.5%. Therefore, the two-year *cumulative incidence of death* of patients after cardiac surgery is 0.535 (1 – 0.465), or 53.5%. The cumulative survival probability is commonly portrayed by a graph, as shown in Figure 3.2.

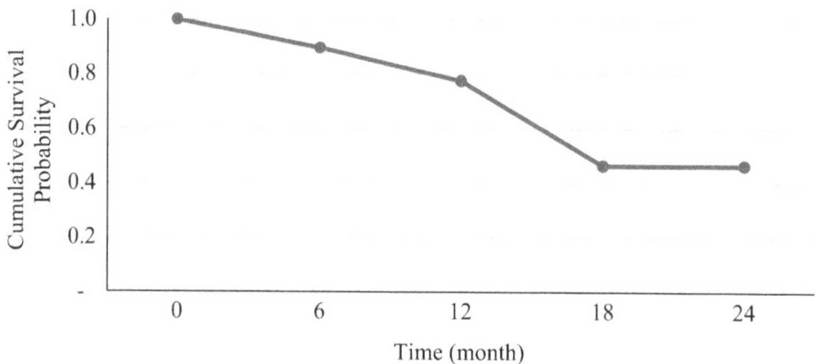

FIGURE 3.2

Cumulative probability of survival after cardiac surgery.

3.2.2.5 Cumulative Incidence: Kaplan-Meier Approach

In contrast to the classic life table approach, the Kaplan-Meier method does not use predetermined intervals, such as one month, six months, or one year, to calculate the survival probabilities. In the Kaplan-Meier method, the probability of an event (incidence) is calculated at the point of occurrence of each event. The number of individuals (usually one) who develop the event at that point constitutes the numerator. The denominator is considered the number of persons at risk at the time of the occurrence of that event, including those who developed the event. It is important to note that the denominator does not include the censored observations (i.e., those who were lost to follow-up before that point).

The main differences between the classic life table approach and the Kaplan-Meier method are that in the classic life table approach, the entire follow-up period is divided into smaller time intervals to calculate the survival probability, while in the Kaplan-Meier approach, survival probabilities are calculated at the points where events occur. The second difference is that in the classic life table approach, the denominator includes half of the censored observations, while in the Kaplan-Meier method, censored observations are omitted from the denominator while calculating the survival probabilities.

Let us consider the data from the previous example (Figure 3.1) for estimating the two-year incidence of death (or cumulative survival probability) after cardiac surgery using the Kaplan-Meier method. The data indicate that deaths occurred at three, eight, 14, and 18 months after enrollment in the study. We will therefore calculate the survival probabilities at each of those time points using a working table (Table 3.3).

TABLE 3.3

Working table for the calculation of cumulative survival probability using the Kaplan-Meier method

Time (in months) of event	No. of individuals at risk	No. of events	Probability of event	Probability of survival	Cumulative probability of survival
C1	C2	C3	C4	C5	C6
3	10	1	0.10	0.90	0.90
8	8	1	0.13	0.87	0.78
14	6	1	0.17	0.83	0.65
18	3	1	0.33	0.67	0.44

Calculations:

C4 (Probability of event)	$= (C3 \div C2)$
C5 (Probability of survival)	$= (1 - C4)$
C6 (Cumulative probability of survival)	$= 0.90$ (same as C5) at 3 months
	$= 0.90 \times 0.87$ at 8 months
	$= 0.90 \times 0.87 \times 0.83$ at 14 months
	$= 0.90 \times 0.87 \times 0.83 \times 0.67$ at 18 months

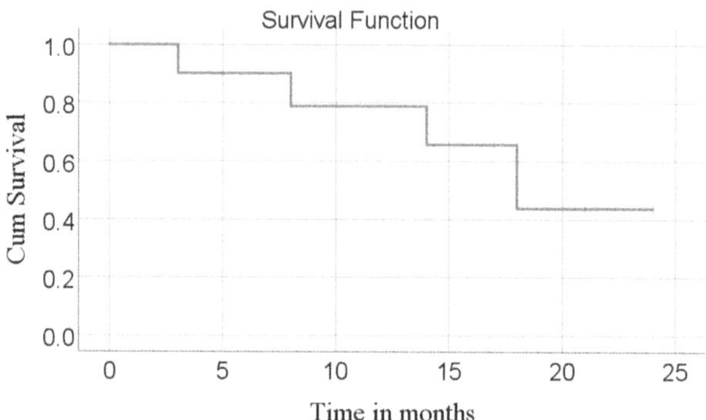

FIGURE 3.3
Cumulative survival probability: Kaplan-Meier method.

The first death (numerator) occurred at three months. At that point, ten persons (including the number of deaths at that point) were at risk of death (denominator). Therefore, the probability (or incidence) of death at three months is 0.10 (1 ÷ 10) and the probability of survival is 0.9 (1 – 0.10).

The second death occurred at eight months. At that point, eight (10 – 2) patients were at risk of death (denominator), as one patient died at three months (patient A), and another was lost to follow-up at five months (patient F). Therefore, the incidence of death at this point is 0.13 (1 ÷ 8) and the survival probability is 0.87 (1 – 0.13). In the same way, we can calculate the probability of events (deaths) and the survival probabilities at 14 and 18 months (Table 3.3).

The cumulative survival probability is calculated in the same manner that we discussed under the classic life table approach (Section 3.4.4). We can use Table 3.3 to work out the two-year cumulative survival probability. In the table, we can see that the cumulative survival probability at 18 months is 0.44. Since there was no more death during the rest of the period, the two-year cumulative survival probability remains the same (0.44) (Figure 3.3). Therefore, the two-year cumulative incidence of death after cardiac surgery is 0.56 (1 – 0.44), or 56.0%. This issue is further discussed in connection with the survival analysis in Chapter 10.

3.3 Incidence Rate: Incidence Based on Person-Time Units at Risk

Person-time is a useful measure for calculating the incidence of outcomes related to morbidity or mortality in many situations, such as in randomized trials and cohort studies. When individuals in a study are observed for different lengths of time (i.e., when all individuals are not observed for the same duration), the person-time of observation (or exposure) is calculated to determine the incidence, referred to as the *incidence rate* (or *incidence density*). The incidence rate indicates how quickly a disease occurs within a population.

Person-time is an estimate of the amount of time the study participants were at risk in the study. An individual contributes person-time to a study as long as she/he is free from the outcome of interest (i.e., still at risk of developing the outcome). The unit of person-time may be the person-year, person-month, or person-day.

Unlike cumulative incidence, the incidence rate is not a proportion. By knowing the number of new cases of a disease and the person-time at risk contributed to the study, an investigator can calculate the incidence rate of that disease. The incidence rate is obtained by dividing the number of new events (disease, deaths, or others) by the amount of person-time observed (at risk) and is measured in units per time.

$$\text{Incidence rate} = \frac{\text{No. of new cases of a disease during a given time period}}{\text{Total person} - \text{time observed}}$$

3.3.1 Incidence Rate Based on Grouped Data

This type of incidence rate is typically calculated for a geographical area by taking the average population (usually the mid-year population) over a certain period of time. Here, the assumption is that losses and events are uniform over the study period and that in- and out-migration are constant. The average population (mid-year population) is calculated by averaging the population at the beginning and end of the study period.

Example

Suppose that there were 2,000 people in a village in January 2020 and 2,100 in December 2021. During this two-year period (2020 and 2021), there were ten deaths in the village. How can we calculate the incidence rate of death for the population?

To calculate the incidence rate of death, we need to calculate the mid-interval population, which is 2,050 [(2,000 + 2,100) ÷ 2]. The amount of time contributed by 2,050 individuals is 4,100 person-years (2,050 × 2 years). Therefore, the incidence rate of death for the population is:

$$\text{Incidence rate of death} = \frac{10}{4,100}$$

$$= 0.0024 \text{ deaths per person} - \text{year,}$$
$$\text{or } 2.4 \text{ deaths per } 1,000 \text{ person} \quad \text{years}$$

3.3.2 Incidence Rate Based on Individual Data

3.3.2.1 Calculating Individual Person-Time of Observation

The first step in measuring the incidence rate for an outcome is to calculate the person-time contributed by each individual in the study. Suppose that an investigator has designed a cohort study to determine the incidence rate of a second heart attack (outcome of interest; case) after an acute heart attack (myocardial infarction or MI). In order to calculate the incidence rate, the researcher followed five individuals (A, B, C, D, and E) from the baseline (from the day of development of the first MI) for a period of 70 days in a hospital. The length of time each patient was observed in this study is graphically presented in Figure 3.4.

The figure shows the number of days each study subject remained in the study as a non-case (did not develop a second heart attack) from the baseline. For example, subject A had a second heart attack on day 20 after the first MI, subject B did not have another heart attack during the entire follow-up period, subject C had a second heart attack on day 29, and so on.

From this information, we can calculate the total person-time contributed by the study subjects to this study. The total person-time observed is the sum of the person-time contributed by each study subject in the study. The unit of the person-time observed in this example is the person-day (p-d). The number of person-days contributed by each study subject is shown below (note that an individual contributes person-time to the study as long as she/ he is free from the outcome of interest):

- Subject A contributed 20 person-days of observation;
- Subject B contributed 70 person-days of observation;
- Subject C contributed 29 person-days of observation;

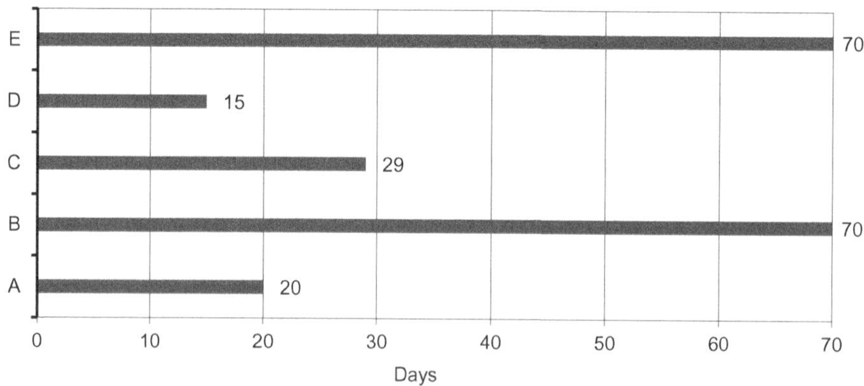

FIGURE 3.4

Follow-up of five patients with myocardial infarction.

- Subject D contributed 15 person-days of observation; and
- Subject E contributed 70 person-days of observation.

The total person-days contributed by all study subjects to this study are 204 person-days (20 + 70 + 29 + 15 + 70). To calculate the incidence rate for a second heart attack, 204 person-days of observation will be the denominator, while the numerator will be the number of subjects who developed the second heart attack (i.e., subjects A, C, and D) during the study period. Therefore, the incidence rate for a second heart attack after the first MI in the study population is:

$$\text{Incidence rate for a second heart attack} =$$

$$\frac{3}{204} = 0.0147 \text{ per person} - \text{day, or } 1.47 \text{ per } 100 \text{ person} - \text{days}$$

The incidence rate can also be expressed in terms of person-months or person-years. In this example, 0.0147 per person-day is equivalent to 5.37 per person-year (we obtained this value by multiplying 0.0147 by 365).

3.3.2.2 Estimating Person-Time When a Person Becomes a Case

Suppose that a researcher is investigating the incidence of breast cancer among women with a family history of breast cancer. To conduct the study, the researcher enrolled five women (A, B, C, D, and E) who had a family history of breast cancer (Figure 3.5). It has been decided to examine the study subjects once a year for up to five years. In order to calculate the person-time for a case when an investigator is only examining individuals at specified intervals (here, once a year), the investigator must decide when the subject acquired the disease. To determine the amount of person-time, it is assumed

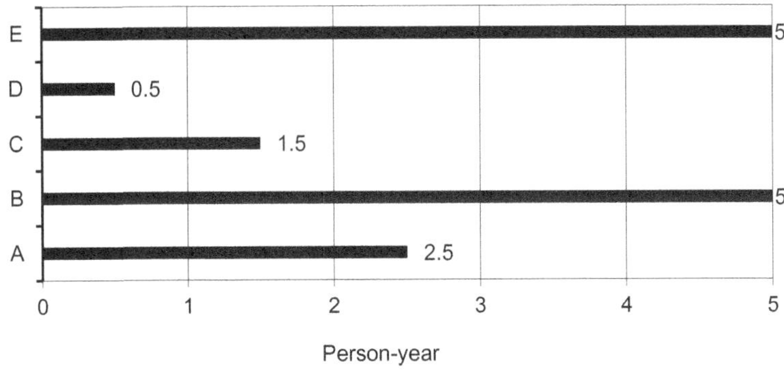

FIGURE 3.5
Follow-up of five women for the detection of breast cancer.

that the disease (breast cancer) occurred at the midpoint of the previous time interval. This is because we do not know precisely when the subject actually developed the disease.

In our example (Figure 3.5), one person (woman D) was diagnosed as a case (breast cancer) in the first follow-up examination (i.e., after one year of follow-up). We will assume that the woman developed the disease in the middle of the first-year follow-up period (first interval), since we do not know exactly when she developed it. Therefore, the woman contributed six months of observation (six person-months) to the study. On the other hand, woman A was disease-free for up to two follow-up periods (two years), and she was found to have breast cancer during the third follow-up visit. The woman, therefore, contributed 2.5 person-years of observation (two years plus 0.5 years) to the study.

Figure 3.5 displays the number of person-years contributed by the study subjects, including the women who developed breast cancer (A, C, and D) during the study period. In this example, the number of person-years contributed by each woman is:

- Woman A: 2.5 person-years of observation;
- Woman B: 5.0 person-years of observation;
- Woman C: 1.5 person-years of observation;
- Woman D: 0.5 person-years of observation; and
- Woman E: 5.0 person-years of observation.

The total person-years of observation contributed by all women to this study are 14.5 (2.5 + 5.0 + 1.5 + 0.5 + 5.0) person-years (denominator). Therefore, the incidence rate of breast cancer is:

$$\text{Incidence rate of breast cancer} =$$

$$\frac{3}{14.5} = 0.207 \text{ per person} - \text{year, or } 20.7 \text{ per } 100 \text{ person} - \text{years}$$

The person-time concept has several concerns [2, 3, 6]. First, a given amount of person-time can be derived from a variety of different circumstances. For instance, the observation of 20 subjects for one year, ten subjects for two years, or five subjects for four years will give the same amount of person-time of observation, and the actual number of people observed in the study cannot be assumed from the data.

Second, the person-time concept assumes that the risk of developing the outcome of interest (disease or death) remains constant throughout the study period, which is often not valid. For example, the risk of death following an acute heart attack (myocardial infarction) is not constant over time; it is highest immediately after the attack, remains elevated for up to 48 hours, and then gradually declines. In situations like this, it is useful to divide the person-time contributed by study subjects into several intervals and calculate the incidence rate separately for each interval.

Third, the person-time concept assumes that the risk of the outcome of interest is the same among individuals lost to follow-up and those who are still under observation, which may not be valid.

Fourth, it is assumed that individuals were lost to follow-up uniformly over the entire study period.

3.4 Relationship Between Cumulative Incidence and Incidence Rate

The cumulative incidence can be estimated from the incidence rate (IR). Suppose that the incidence rate of oral cancer among smokers is 0.00375 per person-year, found in a cohort study. The cumulative incidence of oral cancer among smokers can be estimated from the incidence rate by using the following formula:

$$\text{Cumulative incidence} = 1 - e^{-(\text{IR} \times t)}$$

Where IR represents the incidence rate and t represents the length of follow-up or time period to estimate the cumulative incidence.

Example
Suppose that you want to estimate the ten-year cumulative incidence of oral cancer among smokers from the incidence rate of 0.00375 per person-year. Using the above formula, the estimated ten year cumulative incidence of oral cancer among smokers is:

$$= 1 - e^{-(0.00375 \times 10)} = 0.0368 \text{ or } 3.68\%$$

3.5 Frequently Used Measures of Morbidity and Mortality

In epidemiology, morbidity and mortality indicators are measured to assess the extent of the problem, for comparison, and for decision-making. Table 3.4 shows the numerator, denominator, and constant (multiplier) for the calculation of commonly used morbidity and mortality measures in epidemiology.

　　　　　　　　　　　　　　　　　　Basic Principles of Epidemiology

TABLE 3.4

Calculation of common morbidity and mortality indicators

Indicator	Numerator	Denominator	Constant
Crude death rate (CDR)	Total no. of deaths (irrespective of age, sex, or other characteristics) during a specified year (or period) in a geographical area	Mid-year population of the geographical area during the same year (time period)	1,000
Age-specific death rate	No. of deaths in a specified age group during a given time interval	Mid-interval population in the same age-group	1,000
Sex-specific death rate	No. of deaths in a specified sex group during a given time interval	Mid-interval population of the same sex	1,000
Cause-specific death rate	No. of deaths from a specified cause (e.g., cancer) during a given time interval	Mid-interval population	1,000 or 100,000
Proportional mortality ratio	No. of deaths due to a specified cause (e.g., heart disease) during a given time interval	Total no. of deaths from all causes during the same time interval	100
Proportional mortality ratio for people 60 years and above	No. of deaths of individuals 60 years and above during a given time interval	Total no. of deaths during the same time interval	100
Case fatality rate	No. of deaths from a specified disease during a given time interval	Total no. of cases reported of that disease during the same time interval	100
Neonatal mortality rate (NMR)	No. of neonatal deaths (deaths during 0 to 28 days of life) in a specified time period	No. of live births during the same time period	1,000
Early neonatal mortality rate	No. newborn deaths under 7 days of age reported during a given time interval	No. of live births during the same time interval	1,000
Post-neonatal mortality rate	No. of deaths among children 29–364 days of age during a given time interval	No. of live births during the same time period	1,000
Infant mortality rate (IMR)	No. of infant deaths (<1 year of age) in a specified time period	No. of live births during the same time period	1,000
Child mortality rate	No. of deaths of children aged 1–4 years during a given year (period)	Total no. of children aged 1–4 years at the middle of the year (period)	1,000
Under 5 mortality rate (U5MR)	No. of deaths of children less than 5 years of age in a specified time period	No. of live births during the same time period	1,000
Fetal death rate	No. of fetal deaths (more than 28 weeks of gestation) during a given time interval	No. of fetal deaths plus no. of live births during the same time interval	1,000

TABLE 3.4 (Continued)

Calculation of common morbidity and mortality indicators

Indicator	Numerator	Denominator	Constant
Perinatal mortality rate	No. of fetal deaths (more than 28 weeks of gestation) plus no. of infant deaths up to 7 days of life during a given time interval	No. of fetal deaths plus no. of live births during the same time interval	1,000
Maternal mortality ratio (MMR)	No. of maternal deaths in a specified time period	No. of live births during the same time period	100,000
Maternal mortality rate	No. of maternal deaths in a specified area at specified time interval	Total no. of women at reproductive age (15-49 years) in the same area at mid-time interval	100,000
Crude birth rate (CBR)	Total no. of births (live and stillbirths) during a specified year in a geographical area	Mid-year population of the geographical area during the same year	1,000
Maternal case fatality rate (CFR)	No. of maternal deaths in a health facility (not in the community) in a year (or a specified period)	Total no. of obstetric complications treated in the same facility in the same year (or same period)	100
Contraceptive prevalence rate (CPR)	No. of eligible couple using contraceptive at a particular point in time	Total no. of eligible couple in the area at the same point in time	100
General fertility rate (GFR)	No. of live births in an area during a year	No. of mid-year female population of 15-49 years in the same area	1,000
Met need for emergency obstetric care (EmOC)	No. of pregnancy complications treated at EmOC facilities	Total no. of expected pregnancy complications (15% of expected pregnancies) in the community during the same time period	100
Population growth rate	No. of population increased in a community or country in a year	Total no. of population in the community or country at the beginning of the year	100
Attack rate (usually used in outbreak)	No. of people who developed the disease	Total no. of people of at risk	100
Secondary attack rate	No. of people who developed disease after exposure to the primary case	Total no. of people who were exposed to the primary case	100

3.6 Standardization of Rates: Comparison of Mortality in different Populations

Comparison of basic health indicators is a fundamental aspect of health situation analysis in epidemiology. Crude rates, whether they represent mortality, morbidity, or other health events, are summary measures of population experiences. An important use of mortality or morbidity data is to compare rates to measure differences between two or more populations or in the same population at different time intervals.

The crude rate (e.g., crude death rate) is an overall estimate of an event. It does not take into account possible factors influencing the rate, such as age, socio-economic status, ethnicity, or other factors. Commonly available crude rates (e.g., crude death rates) for various populations or countries may not be directly comparable due to the influence of age structure or other factors. It is, therefore, necessary to standardize crude rates before making a meaningful comparison. There are two different approaches to standardizing rates: the direct method and the indirect method of standardization [3, 11, 12].

3.6.1 Direct Method of Standardization

Table 3.5 (hypothetical data) shows that the crude (overall) death rates for countries A (a developed country) and B (a developing country) in 2000 were 6.02 and 5.93 per 1,000 population, respectively. Looking at these rates, one may erroneously conclude that death rates for countries A and B are almost the same. Typically, the death rate in a developing country is expected to be higher than in a developed country. However, data show that the crude death rates of these two countries are nearly identical, which might be surprising.

One key factor that may influence the crude death rate (CDR) is the age structure (distribution) of the population. Tables 3.6 and 3.7 display the population age structures of two countries. The tables show that in Country B, there are more people in the under-five age group and fewer people in the above-60 age group compared to Country A. This indicates that the age-specific population structures are different in these two countries. For instance, the proportion of the total population above 60 is 19.9% in Country A, compared to 5.6% in Country B. Similarly, the under-five population in

TABLE 3.5

Crude (overall) death rates of countries A and B in 2000

	Country A	Country B
Total population	22,100,000	24,800,000
Total number of deaths	132,950	147,090
Crude (overall) death rates	6.02 deaths per 1,000	5.93 deaths per 1,000

TABLE 3.6

Population structure of Country A with the annual number of deaths and age-specific death rates

Age group	Population (in million)	% of total population	Annual no. of deaths	Age specific death rate per 1,000
<5	1,500,000	6.8	15,620	10.41
5 to 19	4,300,000	19.5	6,530	1.52
20 to 39	7,600,000	34.4	5,620	0.74
40 to 59	4,300,000	19.5	29,690	6.90
60 to 79	3,400,000	15.4	45,350	13.34
≥ 80	1,000,000	4.5	30,140	30.14
Total:	22,100,000	100.0	132,950	6.02

TABLE 3.7

Population structure of Country B with the annual number of deaths and age-specific death rates

Age group	Population	% of total population	Annual no. of deaths	Age specific death rate per 1,000
<5	3,900,000	15.7	49,650	12.73
5 to 19	7,600,000	30.6	20,160	2.65
20 to 39	8,600,000	34.7	10,230	1.19
40 to 59	3,300,000	13.3	25,630	7.77
60 to 79	1,000,000	4.0	22,630	22.63
≥ 80	400,000	1.6	18,790	46.98
Total:	24,800,000	100.0	147,090	5.93

Country A is 6.8%, while it is 15.7% in Country B. It is well documented that mortality rates are usually higher in the under-five and over-60 age groups. As such, an imbalance in population structures can substantially affect the CDR. To address this problem, rates are standardized (or adjusted) before comparisons are made.

Tables 3.6 and 3.7 show the distributions of population by age group and the corresponding number of deaths for two populations. In the direct method of standardization, the population differences in different age groups are eliminated by using a hypothetical population called the "standard population". The standard population is used to make the population composition of each age group the same for both countries. The idea is to nullify the effect of varying population sizes in different age groups on the crude death rates in both countries.

The standard population can be any population, and the selection is somewhat arbitrary. However, there are several options available for choosing a standard population for standardization, such as an entirely hypothetical population, the sum of the study populations, the population of one of the study groups, the population of a state or a country, or the minimum-variance standard population [6]. In our example, we used the standard population as the sum of the study populations (Country A + Country B) in each age category of both countries. For instance, the standard population for the under-five age group is 5,400,000 (1,500,000 + 3,900,000). Similarly, age-specific standard populations are generated for other age groups, as shown in Table 3.8.

Using the age-specific death rate and the standard population, the expected number of deaths for each age group is calculated. This is done by multiplying the age-specific standard population by the corresponding age-specific death rate (in our example, it is per 1,000 population). The expected number of deaths in all age groups is then totaled and divided by the total standard population to get the age-adjusted death rates for both countries (Table 3.8). The age-adjusted death rates represent the rates if both countries had the same age structure.

TABLE 3.8

Age-specific death rates, standard population, and expected number of deaths in countries A and B

Age group	Age-specific death rate per 1,000		Standard population (Population A + B)	Expected no. of deaths	
	Country A	Country B		Country A	Country B
	C1	C2	C3	(C1×C3)/1,000	(C2×C3)/1,000
<5	10.41	12.73	5,400,000	56,214	68,742
5 to 19	1.52	2.65	11,900,000	18,088	31,535
20 to 39	0.74	1.19	16,200,000	11,988	19,278
40 to 59	6.90	7.77	7,600,000	52,440	59,052
60 to 79	13.34	22.63	4,400,000	58,696	99,572
≥ 80	30.14	46.98	1,400,000	42,196	65,772
Total			**46,900,000**	**239,622**	**343,951**

$$\text{Age} - \text{adjusted (standardized) death rate} = \frac{\text{Total expected deaths}}{\text{Total standard population}} \times 1,000$$

$$\text{Age} - \text{adjusted death rate for Country A} = \frac{239,622}{46,900,000} \times 1,000 = 5.11 \text{ per } 1,000$$

$$\text{Age} - \text{adjusted death rate for Country B} = \frac{343,951}{46,900,000} \times 1,000 = 7.33 \text{ per } 1,000$$

Comparative mortality index, CMI

$$= \frac{\text{Standardized death rate for B}}{\text{Standardized death rate for A}} \text{ or } \frac{7.33}{5.11} = 1.43$$

Through this process, the effect of different age distributions of the two countries is adjusted, making the rates comparable. Like age adjustment, rates can be adjusted for other factors, such as sex, socioeconomic status, and race.

Table 3.8 shows that the age-adjusted (age-standardized) death rates for countries A and B are 5.11 and 7.33 per 1,000 population, respectively. The results indicate a higher death rate in Country B compared to Country A, as expected. The comparative mortality index (CMI) calculated from the data is 1.43, indicating that the death rate in Country B is 1.43 times (or 43%) higher than in Country A. It is important to note that adjusted rates are used for the purpose of comparison and do not represent the actual death rates of populations.

3.6.2 Indirect Method of Standardization

When the age-specific mortality rates of one population (or country) are not available but the total number of deaths or crude death rate is available, the indirect method of standardization is used. In this method, the standardized mortality ratio (SMR) is calculated.

$$\text{Standardized mortality ratio, SMR} = \frac{\text{No. of observed deaths}}{\text{No. of expected deaths}}$$

Suppose we want to compare the mortality rates of two countries (or populations): Country A and Country C. The age structure and the age-specific death rates of Country A are available, as shown in Table 3.6. For Country C, only the age-specific population and crude death rate (or total number of observed deaths) are available, as shown in Table 3.9. In the indirect method of standardization, the age-specific death rates of Country A are applied to Country C to calculate the expected number of deaths in each age group (Table 3.10). Table 3.10 shows that the total number of expected deaths in Country C when the age-specific death rates of Country A are applied

TABLE 3.9

Population structure and total number of annual deaths in Country C

Age group	Population	Annual no. of deaths	Age specific death rate per 1,000
<5	2,900,000	Not available	Not available
5 to 19	7,500,000	Not available	Not available
20 to 39	8,200,000	Not available	Not available
40 to 59	3,000,000	Not available	Not available
60 to 79	1,000,000	Not available	Not available
≥ 80	500,000	Not available	Not available
Total:	**23,100,000**	**130,483**	
Crude death rate: 5.65 per 1,000			

TABLE 3.10

Expected number of deaths and SMR for Country C

Age group	Population C	Age-specific death rate of population A (per 1,000)	Expected no. of deaths for population B
<5	2,900,000	10.41	30,189
5 to 19	7,500,000	1.52	11,400
20 to 39	8,200,000	0.74	6,068
40 to 59	3,000,000	6.90	20,700
60 to 79	1,000,000	13.34	13,340
≥ 80	500,000	30.14	15,070
Total:	**23,100,000**		**96,767**

Standardized mortality ratio, SMR is (130,483 ÷ 96,767) or 1.35

is 96,767, while the observed number of deaths was 130,483. Therefore, the standardized mortality ratio (SMR) is 1.35 (130,483 ÷ 96,767).

An SMR value of one indicates that the observed number of deaths is equal to the expected number. If it is more than one, it indicates there are more deaths than expected, while if it is less than one, it is less than the expected number of deaths. In our example, an SMR of 1.35 indicates that the risk of dying for population C is 1.35 times (or 35%) higher than expected according to the mortality standards of population A after adjusting for age. If the SMR were less than one (say, 0.70), it would indicate that population C is 30% less $(1 - 0.7)$ likely to die than expected according to the mortality standards of population A after adjusting for age. SMR is commonly calculated in occupational studies to answer the question, "Do people working in a certain industry have a higher mortality rate than the general population of the same age group?"

3.6.2.1 Confidence Interval for SMR

The confidence interval provides a range of values within which the true (actual) value of the indicator lies in the population with a given probability. The 95% confidence interval (CI) is the most commonly used measure in statistics. The 95% CI indicates the range of values within which we expect to find the true value of the indicator in the study population, with a probability of 95%. The 95% CI for SMR can be calculated using the following formula:

$$95\% \text{ CI of SMR} = \text{SMR} \pm 1.96 \times \left(\text{Standard error of SMR}\right)$$

The standard error (SE) of SMR is calculated as:

$$\text{SE of SMR} = \frac{\text{SMR}}{\sqrt{\left(\text{No. of observed deaths}\right)}}$$

Or,

$$\text{SE of SMR} = \frac{\sqrt{\left(\text{No. of observed deaths}\right)}}{\text{Expected no. of deaths}}$$

In our example, the SE of SMR is:

$$\text{SE of SMR} = \frac{1.35}{\sqrt{130,483)}} = 0.0037$$

Therefore, the 95% CI for SMR is:

$$95\% \text{ CI of SMR} = 1.35 \pm 1.96 \times 0.0037 = 1.34 \text{ to } 1.36$$

In our example, the 95% CI for SMR is 1.34 to 1.36. This indicates that there is a 95% probability that the actual value of SMR will be between 1.34 and 1.36.

Crude rates represent the actual occurrence of events in the population and are important in public health. They provide information about the extent of the problem and the need for resource allocation for health interventions. Although crude rates are easy to calculate, they are confounded by differences in underlying population structures and other factors. Category-specific rates, however, are not affected by these factors. On the other hand, adjusted rates provide summary values after removing the effect of differences in the population structure or other factors, allowing for valid comparisons between groups or over time.

References

1. Mausner JS, Kramer S. *Epidemiology: An Introductory Text.* 2nd ed. Philadelphia: WB Saunders; 1983.
2. Hennekens CH, Buring JE. *Epidemiology in Medicine.* Boston: Little Brown and Company; 1987.
3. Gordis L. *Epidemiology.* 5th ed. Philadelphia: Elsevier Saunders; 2014.
4. Centers for Disease Control and Prevention. *Principles of Epidemiology in Public Health Practice: An Introduction to Applied Epidemiology and Biostatistics.* 3rd ed. Lesson 3: measures of risk; 2022. Available from: file:///C:/Users/HP/Downloads/cdc_6914_DS1.pdf
5. Centers for Disease Control and Prevention (CDC). *Lesson 3: Measures of Risk, Section 2: Morbidity Frequency Measures.* Atlanta, GA: CDC; 2012. Available from:https://archive.cdc.gov/www_cdc_gov/csels/dsepd/ss1978/lesson3/section2.html

6.   Szklo M, Nieto FJ. *Epidemiology: Beyond the Basics.* 2nd ed. Boston: Jones and Bartlett; 2007.

7.   Persson LA, Wall S. *Epidemiology for Public Health.* Sweden: Umea University; 2000.

8.   Noordzij M, Dekker FW, Zoccali C, Jager KJ. Measures of disease frequency: prevalence and incidence. *Nephron Clin Pract.* 2010;115:c17–20. doi: 10.1159/000286345

9.   Jager KJ, Zoccali C, Kramar R, Dekker FW. Measuring disease occurrence. *Kidney Int.* 2007;72:412–5. doi: 10.1038/sj.ki.5002341

10. National Institute of Preventive and Social Medicine (NIPSOM). *National STEPS Survey for Non-Communicable Diseases Risk Factors in Bangladesh.* Bangladesh: Ministry of Health and Family Welfare; 2018.

11. Lilienfeld DE, Stolley PD. *Foundations of Epidemiology.* 3rd ed. New York: Oxford University Press; 1994.

12. Naing NN. Easy way to learn standardization: Direct and indirect methods. *Malays J Med Sci.* 2000;7(1):10–15.

4

Epidemiological Study Designs: An Overview

Mohammad Tajul Islam

The primary objective of epidemiology is to assess the relationship between exposure and disease (or any other outcome). To assess the relationship, the researcher first identifies a research question and defines the hypothesis. Based on the research question and hypothesis, the researcher decides which study design will best answer the research question. Epidemiological study designs are a set of methods and procedures that are used to collect and analyze data on diseases or health-related problems to answer one or more research questions. Basic concepts and types of epidemiological study designs, including their advantages and limitations, are discussed in this chapter. Details about the study designs are discussed in subsequent chapters.

4.1 Types of Epidemiological Studies

Epidemiological studies can be broadly classified into descriptive studies and analytic studies (Figure 4.1) [1–3].

4.1.1 Descriptive Studies

Descriptive studies are usually undertaken when little is known about the epidemiology of a disease. Descriptive studies are designed primarily to describe the distribution of a disease in the community. Descriptive studies describe the disease patterns and their extent and severity in the community. In descriptive studies, the patterns of disease occurrence, such as variations in disease frequency among populations by individual characteristics (person), geographical areas (place), and over time (time), are described [1, 4]. The primary difference between descriptive and analytic studies is that descriptive studies do not test hypotheses, whereas analytic studies are

DOI: 10.1201/9781003654803-4

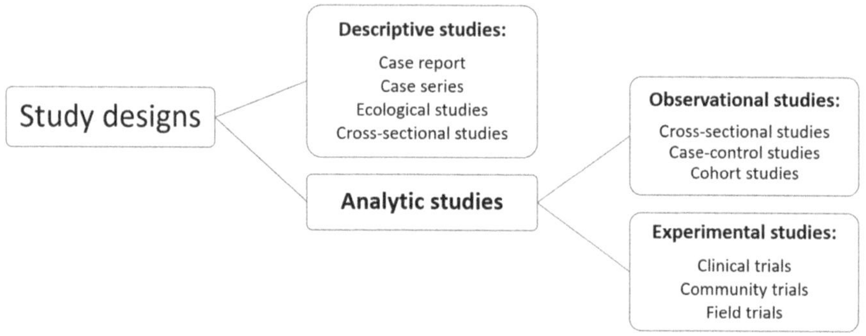

FIGURE 4.1
Epidemiological study designs.

designed to test them. However, descriptive studies are helpful in generating research questions and hypotheses that are tested in analytic study designs. Descriptive studies include:

a. Case reports;
b. Case series;
c. Ecological or correlational studies; and
d. Cross-sectional studies.

4.1.2 Analytic Studies

Analytic studies are conducted to identify the risk factor(s) for a disease or evaluate interventions for the control of a disease or a health-related problem. Analytic studies are concerned with testing hypotheses about exposure and outcome. For hypothesis testing, an appropriate comparison group is needed. Analytic studies can be divided into two broad categories:

a. Observational studies, such as cross-sectional, case-control, and cohort studies; and
b. Experimental studies, such as intervention trials (clinical trials, community trials, and field trials).

4.1.2.1 Observational Studies

In observational studies, the investigator simply observes the natural course of events. In this design, exposure is not under the control of the investigator. Individuals are exposed spontaneously. The investigator observes only the groups that are naturally exposed or unexposed to the putative factor, as well as the occurrence of the disease of interest in these groups. Statistical methods are then applied to determine whether an association exists between the exposure and the disease [1, 5, 6]. The observational studies include:

a. Cross-sectional studies;
b. Case-control studies; and
c. Cohort studies.

4.1.2.2 Experimental Studies

Experimental studies are commonly done to evaluate the effectiveness of an intervention program, such as the impact of an intervention for the prevention of a disease or the efficacy of a drug on disease outcomes. In experimental studies, exposure is under the control of the investigator (i.e., the investigator decides and allocates the exposure). The investigator assigns exposure to a group (or groups) of people, follows them for a certain period of time, and observes the occurrence of the outcome [1, 2, 6, 7].

Experimental studies can be randomized or non-randomized [5, 6]. In randomized designs, intervention (exposure) is assigned to study subjects (or communities) randomly, i.e., who will (or will not) receive the intervention is decided through a random process. In non-randomized trials, the intervention (exposure) is not assigned to the subjects or communities randomly, i.e., the intervention is decided based on a non-random process, such as convenience or judgment. The non-randomized trials are called *quasi-experimental* designs. When an experimental study has a comparison group, it is called a controlled trial, e.g., a randomized controlled trial (RCT). Of all epidemiological study designs, randomized controlled trials are often considered the gold standard [6]. Experimental studies can be:

> *Clinical trials:* In clinical trials, an intervention is provided to individuals with a disease to evaluate the impact of the intervention, such as a drug trial at a hospital. For example, Alam et al. (1990) conducted a randomized double-blind study to compare the efficacy of a single dose of doxycycline with the standard multiple doses of tetracycline in patients with cholera. The study concluded that a single dose of doxycycline is as effective as the standard multiple doses of tetracycline for the treatment of cholera in adults [8].

> *Community trials:* In community trials, intervention is undertaken for the community as a whole, e.g., health education to pregnant women in a community to assess its impact on utilization of healthcare services. For instance, Trobe et al. (2019) conducted a community-based cluster randomized trial in an Upazila (sub-district) in Bangladesh. The clusters were randomly allocated to either receive the intervention (health education for pregnant women) or no intervention (control group). The

study found that health education to pregnant women was effective in improving utilization of maternal healthcare services [9].

Field trials: In field trials, preventive interventions are applied to healthy individuals who are at risk of developing a disease, e.g., a vaccine trial. Data collection in field trials takes place in the field, usually in the general population [7].

4.2 Descriptive Study Designs

4.2.1 Case Report

This is the most basic type of descriptive study design. Such studies describe the experience of a single case. The investigator carefully prepares a detailed report describing the profile of a single patient. The advantages and limitations of case reports are described in Table 4.1.

4.2.2 Case Series

In a case series, the experience of a number of cases with a similar disease is described. The case series may provide clues to the beginning of the emergence of an epidemic. The advantages and limitations of case series are provided in Table 4.2.

4.2.3 Ecological Studies

Ecological studies are also called correlational studies. In ecological studies, data on exposure and outcome are not collected from individuals. They are collected at group levels. Such studies utilize data already available (secondary data) from the entire population to compare disease frequencies among groups during the same time period (cross-sectional ecological studies) or within the same population at different points in time (time-trend ecological studies). Since data are not collected from individuals, the results

TABLE 4.1

Advantages and limitations of case reports

Advantages	Limitations
• Simple, inexpensive, and can be conducted within a short period of time • Help in generating research questions and hypotheses • May provide an initial clue of the emergence of a new disease or an unusual adverse event of a drug	• Although case reports can help generate hypotheses, they cannot be tested within this study design

TABLE 4.2

Advantages and limitations of case series

Advantages	Limitations
• Case series are simple, inexpensive, and can be conducted within a short period of time • Help in generating research questions and hypotheses • May provide initial clues to the emergence of an epidemic in the community	• Case series help in generating hypotheses but cannot test them due to the lack of a comparison group

TABLE 4.3

Advantages and limitations of ecological studies

Advantages	Limitations
• Since correlational studies utilize pre-existing data, they can be conducted with minimal time and resources • They help in generating hypotheses about associations between exposure and disease	• Correlational studies present average values of exposure rather than actual exposure at the individual level • In correlational studies, data are collected from populations as a whole rather than from individuals. It is therefore not possible to link exposure directly to disease occurrence at the individual level • If an association is found between an exposure and a disease, the study cannot confirm causation • Such studies are subjected to confounding bias that cannot be adjusted for during analysis

of ecological studies are applicable only at the population level. Such studies cannot confirm the causal relationship between exposure and outcome but help in generating hypotheses (see Table 4.3) [1, 2, 4].

4.2.4 Cross-Sectional Studies

Cross-sectional studies are also called prevalence surveys. In this study design, the status of individuals' exposure and outcome are measured at the same point in time. Since exposure and outcome are measured at the same point in time, it may not be possible to determine the temporal relationship between exposure and outcome (i.e., whether exposure preceded or followed the development of the disease). This study design is typically used to determine the prevalence of a disease and its distribution within a population (a descriptive cross-sectional study). A cross-sectional study can also be analytic, where associations between exposures and disease are assessed using inferential statistics (analytic cross-sectional study) [1, 2, 10]. The advantages and limitations of cross-sectional studies are described in Table 4.4.

To conduct a cross-sectional study, the investigator takes a representative sample from a population without knowing the exposure and outcome status

TABLE 4.4

Advantages and limitations of cross-sectional studies

Advantages	Limitations
• Cross-sectional studies ca be conducted quickly and easily with limited resources compared to cohort studies • They provide information to understand the disease patterns and extent of the problem in the community, which helps the managers set priorities, allocate resources, and plan for intervention • They are useful to find associations between possible risk factors and disease without the question of temporality, except for permanent characteristics (e.g., sex, race, blood group, and ethnicity) • Help in generating research questions and hypotheses	• They only provide information about disease prevalence, not disease incidence in the community • Provide "snapshot" information about the community at a specific point in time • In most instances, the causal relationship between a factor and disease cannot be determined • Sometimes, it is difficult to infer the temporal relationship between exposure and outcome • Not good for diseases with a short duration and a high case fatality rate • Require a well-planned sampling scheme to generalize the findings • There are problems of non-response in such study designs

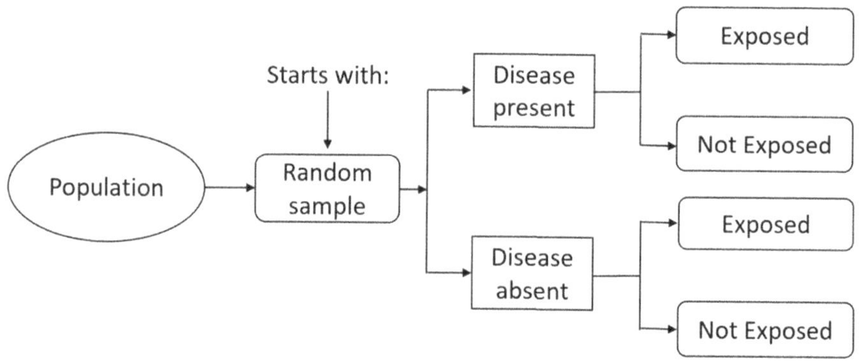

FIGURE 4.2
Cross-sectional study design.

of individuals. Once study subjects are selected, they are classified according to exposure (exposed or unexposed) and disease status (disease present or absent), and the data are analyzed (Figure 4.2).

4.3 Analytic Study Designs

4.3.1 Case-Control Studies

Case-control studies are sometimes called retrospective studies, but this term can be misleading and is best avoided. Case-control studies always start with the outcome of interest. To conduct a case-control study, it is necessary to select a group of people who have the disease (the case) and another group of people who do not have the disease (the control). The researcher then takes the past history of exposure from both groups for comparison, such as the proportion of cases exposed versus the proportion of controls exposed (Figure 4.3). Case-control studies are commonly conducted to identify the risk factors for a disease [1, 2, 10]. The advantages and limitations of case-control studies are provided in Table 4.5.

4.3.2 Cohort Studies

Cohort studies are also called longitudinal, prospective, or follow-up studies. Cohort studies always start with exposure. To conduct a cohort

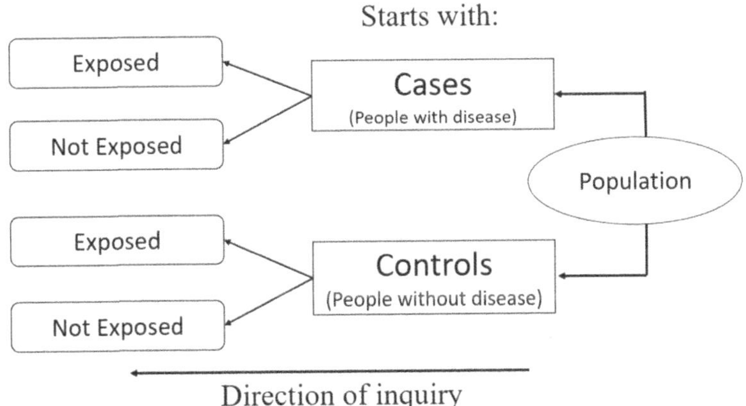

FIGURE 4.3

Case-control study design.

TABLE 4.5

Advantages and limitations of case-control studies

Advantages	Limitations
• Case-control studies are relatively quick and inexpensive compared with other analytic studies • They can be conducted with a small sample size • Suitable for the evaluation of risk factors for a rare disease or disease with a long latent period • Multiple risk (etiology) factors can be studied for a single disease	• The incidence and prevalence rates for a disease cannot be calculated from the data • Not suitable for the evaluation of diseases with rare exposure, unless the exposure rate among cases is high • Cannot directly compute the relative risk. An indirect measure of risk (odds ratio) is calculated • Prone to bias (such as selection, recall, and misclassification bias) compared with other analytic studies • In some situations temporal relationship between exposure and outcome is difficult to ascertain

study, a group of people free from the disease of interest at the beginning is selected who are exposed, and another group (comparison group), also free from the disease of interest, is selected who are not exposed. Both groups are then followed over a certain period of time to observe the occurrence of the outcome (disease of interest) [1, 2, 4]. From cohort study data, one can calculate the incidence and relative risk for a disease. Cohort studies can be classified as:

a.   Prospective or concurrent cohort studies; and

b.   Retrospective, non-concurrent, or historical cohort studies.

In prospective cohort studies, exposed and unexposed groups are followed from the present time to the future (Figure 4.4). In prospective cohort studies, exposures may or may not have occurred, but the outcomes have certainly not yet occurred at the time of the beginning of the study. Therefore, the groups need to be followed in the future.

On the other hand, retrospective cohort studies begin at a time before the present time (Figure 4.5). The investigator identifies a group of people who were exposed in the past and simultaneously selects another group of people who were not exposed. Both groups must be free from the disease of interest at the time of defining the exposure status. In retrospective cohort studies, both exposure and outcome have already occurred when the study is initiated. However, both studies (prospective and retrospective cohort studies) begin with exposure. The advantages and limitations of cohort studies are summarized in Table 4.6.

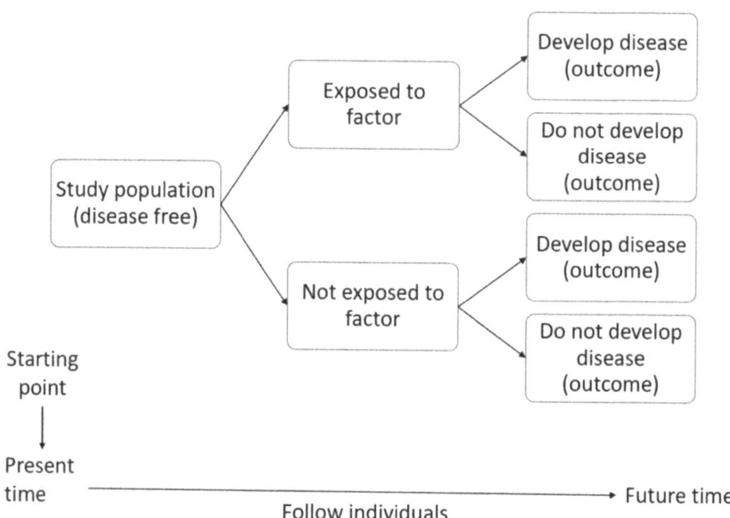

FIGURE 4.4
Prospective or concurrent cohort study design.

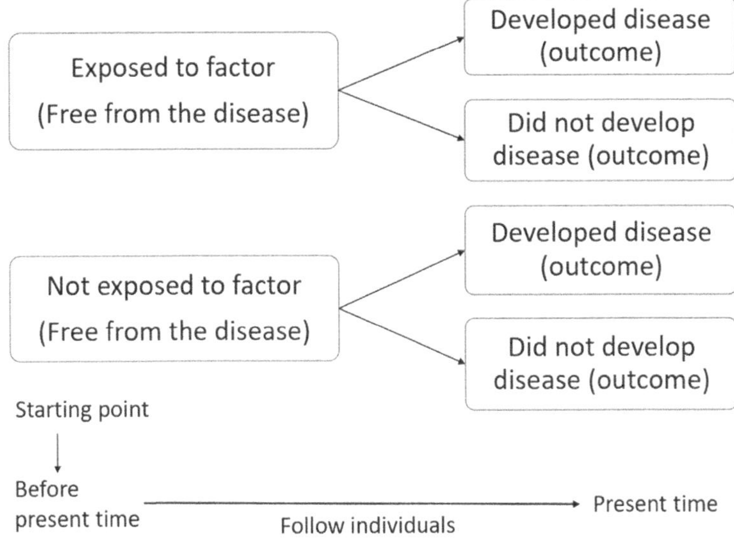

FIGURE 4.5
Retrospective or historical cohort study design.

TABLE 4.6

Advantages and limitations of cohort studies

Advantages	Limitations
• The temporal relationship between exposure and disease can be clearly established	• Cohort studies are generally time consuming and expensive
• This design is most suitable to study rare exposures	• It is necessary to follow a large number of individuals for a long period of time
• Multiple outcomes for a single exposure can be examined	• Cohort studies have a potential bias associated with losses in follow-up
• Tend to minimize the selection bias	• Are inefficient for the evaluation of rare diseases
• Allow to measure the incidence of disease in the exposed and unexposed groups and thus the relative risk	• Retrospective cohort studies require availability of adequate records

4.3.3 Experiential Studies

Experimental (or intervention) studies are broadly a type of cohort study since the studies begin with exposure (commonly an intervention) and follow-up of individuals is needed. Experimental studies are also called trials. Intervention studies (or trials) provide direct evidence of whether an exposure causes or prevents a disease. In intervention studies, the exposure status of each participant (or community) is assigned by the investigator.

As discussed earlier (Section 4.1.2.2), experimental studies can be randomized or non-randomized. Randomization is mainly done to enable

TABLE 4.7

Advantages and limitations of experimental designs

Advantages	Limitations
• Experimental designs provide the most reliable and direct evidence on which to judge whether an exposure causes or prevents a disease • Randomization is a means to make the intervention and comparison groups similar to known and unknown factors that might influence the results	• Ethical concerns preclude the allocation of exposures that are known to be hazardous • Expensive, and sometimes feasibility is a concern • The sample may not be representative • Loss to follow-up and non-compliance may create problems in the interpretation of results

exposed (intervention) and unexposed (non-intervention) groups to be similar to all known and unknown factors. In a randomized controlled trial (RCT), there is one or more comparison or control groups. The experimental group gets the intervention (e.g., a drug, a vaccine, or other intervention), which is expected to be associated with the prevention or better outcome of a disease. The comparison group receives either no treatment, a placebo treatment, or another standard treatment, depending on the study objective. The groups are then followed prospectively to observe who develops the outcome of interest. The advantages and limitations of experimental studies are described in Table 4.7.

4.4 Hierarchy of Study Designs

Epidemiological studies are used to generate evidence about the causal relationship between an exposure and an outcome. The study design and the outcome measured in a study can affect the strength of the evidence. To ensure validity, study results need to be unbiased. A hierarchy (or level) of study designs is a ranking system used to describe the relative strength of study designs, considering the probability of bias.

Of the epidemiological study designs, randomized controlled trials (RCTs) are considered the gold standard, i.e., given the highest level, because they are most likely to be unbiased. On the contrary, ecological studies are at the bottom of the hierarchy because they are most likely to be biased [11]. The relative strength of epidemiological study designs is shown in Figure 4.6.

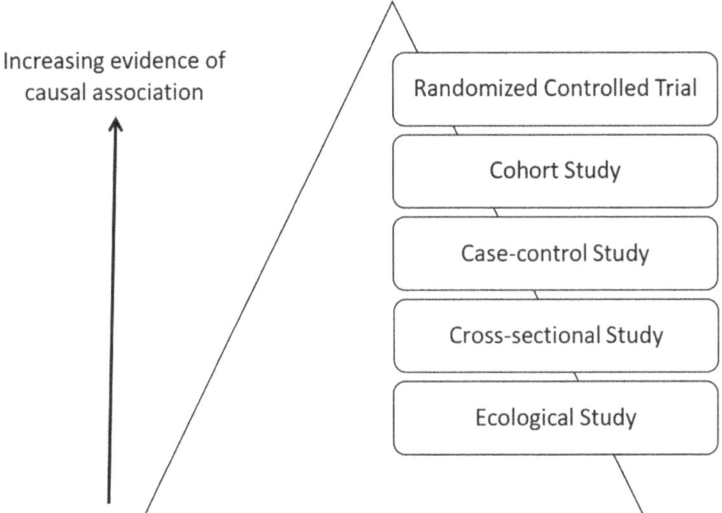

FIGURE 4.6
Hierarchy of study designs in assessing causality.

4.5 Choice of Study Designs

Epidemiological study designs have their own strengths and limitations for investigating the relationship between exposure and outcome. Therefore, the study design should be well thought out before conducting a study. The selection of an inappropriate design may fail to answer the research question under investigation or make the study invalid. Critical thinking for selecting a design beforehand is needed to ensure that the design will adequately answer the research question(s) as well as feasible for implementation. The choice of study design to study a particular exposure-outcome relationship depends on:

- Research question and hypothesis to be tested;
- Nature of the disease under investigation: If the disease is rare, a case-control study is preferred;
- Type of exposure: To investigate a rare exposure for an outcome, a cohort study is preferred, provided the incidence of the outcome is high. Cohort studies are also suitable for investigating the relatively common outcome;
- Results of previous studies and gaps in knowledge that need to be answered;

- Ethical considerations: Ethical considerations in research are a set of principles that guide research designs and conductions. Ethical clearance is needed for all kinds of epidemiological studies; and

- Logistic considerations, such as time and resources available for the study.

References

1. Hennekens CH, Buring JE. *Epidemiology in Medicine.* 1st ed. Boston/Toronto: Little Brown and Company; 1987.
2. Gordis L. *Epidemiology.* 5th ed. Philadelphia: Elsevier Saunders; 2014.
3. Checkoway H, Pearce N, Kriebel D. Selecting appropriate study designs to address specific research questions in occupational epidemiology. *Occup Environ Med.* 2007;64:633–8. doi:10.1136/oem.2006.029967
4. Omair A. Selecting the appropriate study design for your research: Descriptive study designs. *J Health Spec.* 2015;3:153–6. doi:10.4103/1658-600X.159892
5. Noordzij M, Dekker FW, Zoccali C, Jager KJ. Study designs in clinical research. *Nephron Clin Pract.* 2009;113(3):c218–21. doi:10.1159/000235610
6. Evans J. Epidemiology in practice: Randomized controlled trials. *Community Eye Health.* 1998;11(26):26–7.
7. Bonita R, Beaglehole R, Kjellström T. *Basic Epidemiology.* 2nd ed. Geneva: World Health Organization; 2006.
8. Alam AN, Alam NH, Ahmed T, Sack DA. Randomized double blind trial of single dose doxycycline for treating cholera in adults. *BMJ.* 1990;300:1619–27. doi: 10.1136/bmj.300.6740.1619
9. Tobe RG, Islam MT, Yoshimura Y, Hossain J. Strengthening the Community Support Group to improve maternal and neonatal health seeking behaviors: A cluster-randomized controlled trial in Satkhira District, Bangladesh. *PLoS One.* 2019;14(3):e0212847. doi:10.1371/journal.pone.0212847
10. DiPietro NA. Methods in epidemiology: Observational study designs. *Pharmacotherapy.* 2010;30(10):973–84. doi:10.1592/phco.30.10.973
11. Stephenson JM, Babiker A. Overview of study design in clinical epidemiology. *Sex Transm Infect.* 2000;76:244–7. doi:10.1136/sti.76.4.244

5

Descriptive Studies

Mohammad Tajul Islam

Diseases are not uniformly distributed throughout populations. There are variations in the occurrence of diseases among various characteristics of individuals, geographical areas, and over time. When a specific disease is more prevalent in one population than in another or in one country than in another, it helps generate research questions and hypotheses. Epidemiology is primarily concerned with the study of the distribution and determinants of diseases or any health-related problems in the community. Depending on the objective, epidemiological studies for the investigation of health problems can be descriptive or analytic. This chapter discusses different types of descriptive study designs in detail.

5.1 Descriptive Studies

Descriptive studies are epidemiological study designs that describe the patterns of disease occurrence (not the determinants) in a given population. The term "patterns" refers to the distribution of a disease or health-related problem in terms of *person, place, and time*. Descriptive studies answer three basic questions about the occurrence of a disease. They are: who is affected (Who), where the disease occurs (Where), and when the disease occurs (When). The objectives of descriptive studies are to understand the burden and distribution of health problems and to generate research questions and hypotheses [1–7].

Descriptive studies are useful to both health managers and epidemiologists. Health managers use descriptive study findings to understand the extent and severity of health problems, set priorities, efficiently allocate resources, prepare for emergencies (e.g., for epidemics or seasonal fluctuations), and design interventions to control diseases. On the other hand, epidemiologists

DOI: 10.1201/9781003654803-5

utilize information from descriptive studies to formulate research questions and hypotheses, which are then tested in analytic studies.

Descriptive studies, like case reports, case series, and ecological studies, commonly utilize information from available sources, such as hospital clinical records, survey data (e.g., demographic and health surveys), census data, or vital statistics. Additionally, descriptive studies can be conducted by collecting cross-sectional data directly from a population by taking a random sample.

Descriptive studies can be conducted with minimal resources (less expensive) and more quickly than analytic studies. Data from descriptive studies conducted in different populations or at different times in the same population may help identify geographical variations and changes over time in the frequency of a disease. Descriptive epidemiology describes the occurrence of a disease in terms of person, place, and time, as described below.

5.1.1 Person

Descriptive studies analyze data to understand variations in disease frequency in various characteristics of individuals. It has been observed that different personal characteristics of hosts affect the frequency of occurrence and outcome of diseases. Personal characteristics that may affect disease occurrence and outcome include age, sex, race, religion, ethnicity, occupation, socio-economic factors, marital and nutritional status, and other factors. These characteristics are, therefore, included and analyzed in almost all descriptive studies, and data are presented in the form of tables or graphs.

For instance, the occurrence of diarrhea is more common among individuals of low socio-economic status, mainly because of an unhygienic living environment and a lack of safe water supply, proper sanitation (e.g., disposal of sewage), and awareness. The relationship between disease and socio-economic status may also be related to behavioral factors, such as smoking, consumption of alcohol, lack of exercise, and unhealthy food habits. Examples of age and sex as determinants of diseases include measles that occurs in childhood, cancer in middle age, and coronary heart disease in older ages, while diabetes mellitus, hypertension, and obesity are more common in women.

Figure 5.1 shows the age and sex distribution of COVID-19 patients admitted to a hospital in Dhaka. Data indicate that the majority of hospitalized cases were individuals aged between 21 and 60 years, with males being predominantly affected by the infection.

5.1.2 Place

The occurrence of a disease may vary from place to place because of the environmental factors to which individuals are exposed. The place may be the place of residence, workplace, place of recreation, or other places. The

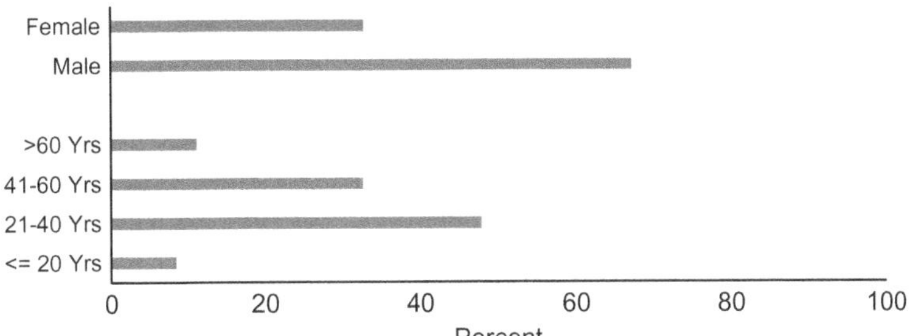

FIGURE 5.1

Distribution of COVID-19 patients admitted to a hospital by age and sex. (Unpublished data from a hospital in Bangladesh.)

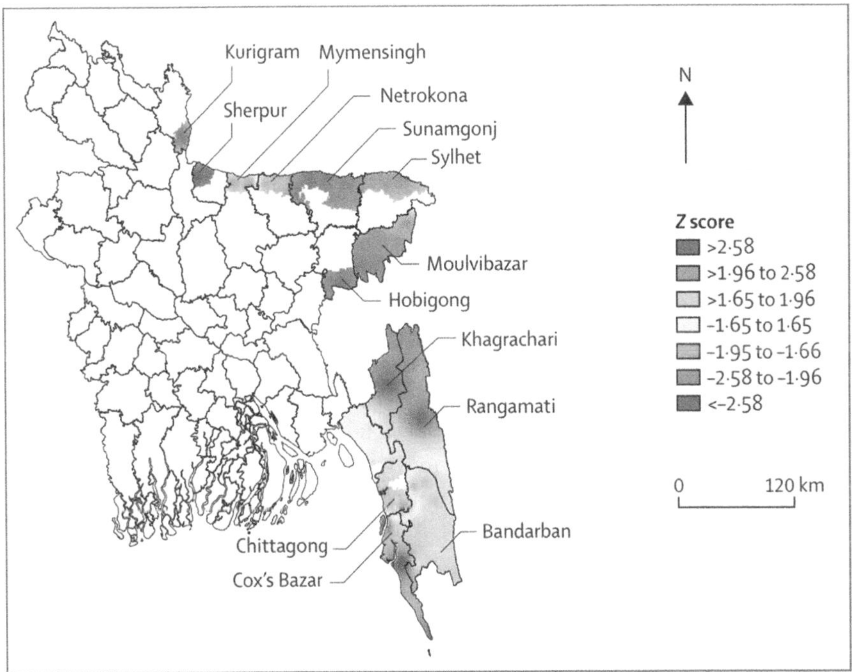

FIGURE 5.2

Malaria-affected districts in Bangladesh. (With the permission from Haque et al. [8].)

distribution of disease occurrence by place provides insights about the extent of the geographical areas affected and its variation among the affected areas. Analyzing data by place helps identify communities at increased risk for a disease. Figure 5.2 shows the endemic areas of malaria in Bangladesh [8]. Malaria is prevalent in 13 of the 64 districts, mainly in the hilly districts bordering India and Myanmar. Comparison of the occurrence of a disease in different places may lead to further investigation of the disease's etiology. The occurrence of a disease may be compared as:

- International comparison, such as comparing across countries (e.g., the incidence of stomach cancer in Japan is four times higher than in the UK [9], and esophageal cancer is more common in Iran than in other regional countries [10]);

- Comparison within the same country, e.g., comparison of the incidence of malaria among districts, and comparison of contraceptive prevalence rates among provinces in Bangladesh;

- Urban-rural comparison, e.g., comparison of the infant mortality rates between urban and rural areas; and

- Local distributions, such as the distribution of a disease in slum and non-slum areas of a city.

The important factors that influence the occurrence of a disease may include population density, level of sanitation (e.g., access to safe water and proper sewerage disposal), air pollution (e.g., the degree of industrialization and the number of vehicles on the streets), the biological environment (e.g., the presence of wild animals, rodents, plants, or bacteria that affect human life), and weather conditions (e.g., rainfall, humidity, and temperature). To assess the geographical extent affected by a disease, data are analyzed by geographical areas and presented as graphs or maps.

5.1.3 Time

The occurrence of a disease usually varies over time. Some of these variations occur regularly, while others are unpredictable. For example, upper respiratory tract infections are more common during the winter months, from November to January. On the other hand, the occurrence of salmonellosis (typhoid and paratyphoid) is unpredictable. For diseases that occur seasonally (e.g., dengue, diarrhea, and influenza) (Figure 5.3) [11], health managers can prepare contingency plans in advance and implement them as needed to prevent outbreaks. In contrast, sporadic diseases often require investigation to identify their causes, risk factors, and modes of transmission before designing effective interventions.

Occurrence of a disease (or a health problem) over time is usually displayed by line graphs or histograms. A line graph is particularly useful to study the trend over time (Figures 5.4 and 5.5) [11, 12] and the effect of interventions from a particular point in time (Figure 5.6) [8], if recorded. Figure 5.6 shows that there has been a steady decline in the prevalence of malaria in Bangladesh from 2008 to 2012 because of interventions. A similar declining trend is also observed in neonatal, infant, and under-five mortality rates in

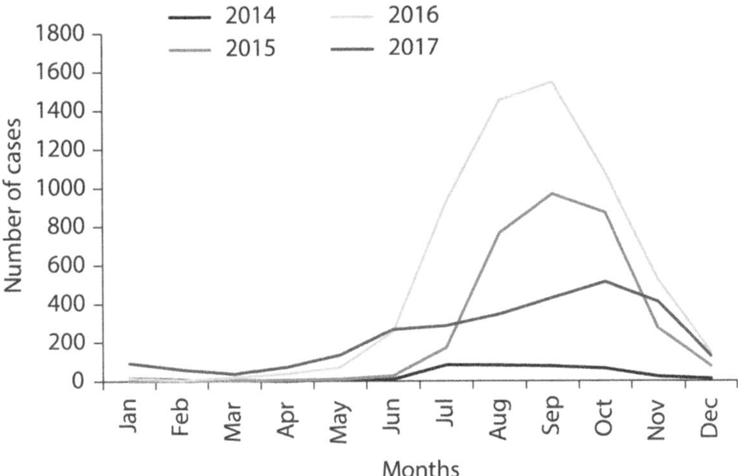

FIGURE 5.3

Seasonal variations of dengue cases in Bangladesh. (With the permission from Mutsuddy et al. [11].)

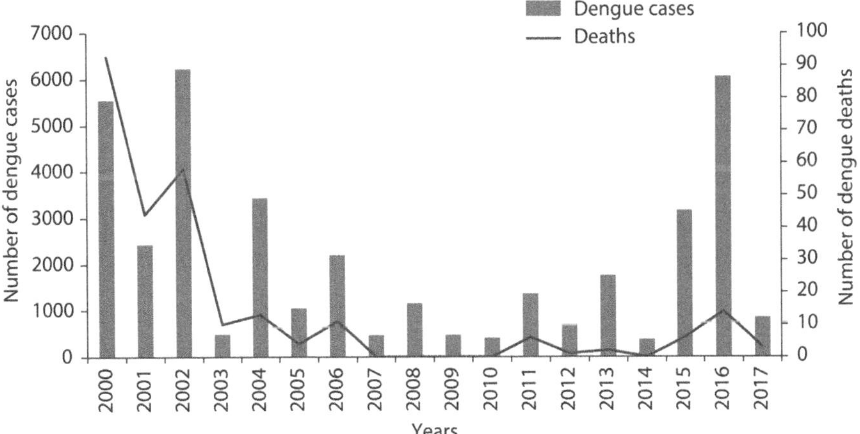

FIGURE 5.4

Secular trend of dengue infections in Bangladesh: 2000–2017. (With the permission from Mutsuddy et al. [11].)

Bangladesh over time, though neonatal mortality has decreased at a slower rate compared to infant and under-five mortality (Figure 5.5). The time trend and fluctuations of disease occurrence over time are described as:

- Long-term fluctuations (secular trend) of diseases like cancer, deaths due to coronary heart disease, diabetes mellitus, neonatal mortality, and malaria;

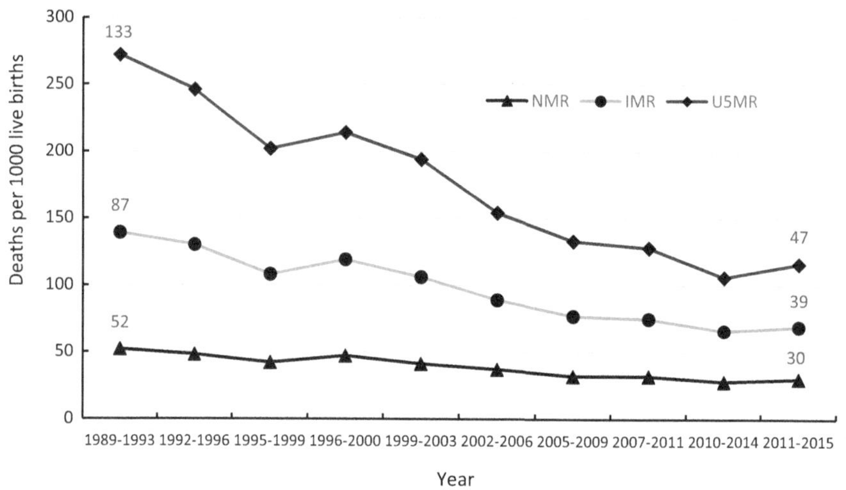

FIGURE 5.5

Trend of neonatal, infant, and under-five mortality rates per 1,000 live births in Bangladesh: 1989–2015. (Drawn with data from the National Institute of Population Research and Training (NIPORT), International Centre for Diarrhoeal Disease Research, Bangladesh (icddr,b), and MEASURE Evaluation. Bangladesh Maternal Mortality and Health Care Survey 2016: Final Report. Dhaka, Bangladesh, and Chapel Hill, NC, USA: NIPORT, icddr,b, and MEASURE Evaluation; 2019.)

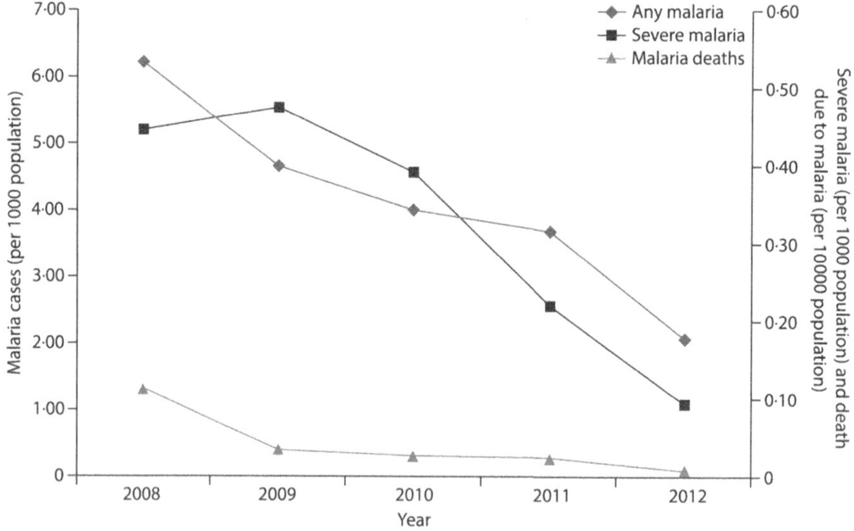

FIGURE 5.6

Prevalence of malaria, severe malaria, and malaria deaths in Bangladesh: 2008–2012. (With the permission from Haque et al. [8].)

- Periodic fluctuations of diseases (or seasonal or cyclic trends), such as measles cases are mostly seen in early spring, upper respiratory tract infections are more prevalent in winter, and dengue occurs more frequently during monsoon and post-monsoon periods; and

- Short-term fluctuations, e.g., fluctuations during an epidemic of a disease.

For long-term trends (also called secular trends), the annual occurrence of a disease is plotted over several years (Figures 5.4 to 5.6). Such graphs are useful for assessing the prevailing trend – whether increasing, decreasing, or stable – and for evaluating the effectiveness of intervention programs. For instance, Figure 5.6 shows a steady decline in the prevalence of malaria in Bangladesh from 2008 to 2012 following the implementation of interventions. This indicates that interventions undertaken by the government were effective.

Disease occurrence can also be graphed by month (or week or day) over the period of a year to study seasonal variations. For example, Figure 5.3 illustrates the seasonal patterns of dengue infection in Bangladesh, showing that dengue cases begin to rise in June and peak in September. Sometimes, displaying data by day or time of day is particularly useful, especially during epidemics (e.g., COVID-19 or dengue epidemics) or when investigating an outbreak of food poisoning.

5.2 Types of Descriptive Studies

Descriptive studies can be of several types, namely, case reports, case series, ecological studies, and cross-sectional studies. In this section, all the descriptive study designs, except for cross-sectional studies, are discussed. The cross-sectional studies are discussed in Chapter 6.

5.2.1 Case Report and Case Series

Case reports and case series are frequently published articles in medical journals. A case report refers to a detailed description of a single patient with an uncommon disease (rare or unfamiliar), an unusual presentation of a common disease, a new adverse effect of a drug, a new technique of investigation, an unexpected event in the course of treating a patient, or an uncommon outcome of a treatment. In case reports, a detailed description of the symptoms, signs, investigations, diagnosis, treatment, follow-up, and outcome is provided.

Case reports can provide the first clues to the emergence of a new disease or the adverse effects of medications. For example, HIV/AIDS was first recognized through a case report of disseminated Kaposi's sarcoma in a young homosexual man [13].

A case series is similar to a case report except that it describes the experiences of a group of patients (often only a few cases) with a similar disease, which may occur in a fairly short period of time. Such studies are important, especially to identify the beginning or presence of an epidemic.

Case reports and case series may lead to the generation of research questions and hypotheses. Although such studies provide important clues for the generation of hypotheses, they cannot be tested because of the lack of a comparison group. Some examples of case reports and case series can be seen elsewhere [14–16]. The advantages and limitations of case reports and case series are described in Chapter 4.

5.2.2 Ecological Studies

Ecological studies are also called correlational studies. Ecological studies are designed to find associations between exposures and outcomes at the population level, not at the individual level. In ecological studies, the unit of observation is a group, not separate individuals.

Since information is not collected from individuals, exposure and risk factors are known only at the group level, such as average coffee consumption (or the proportion of the population who smoke) in different districts (or communities or countries). Similarly, disease occurrence (or mortality) is also known at the group level, such as the incidence of stomach cancer (or cancer deaths or other measures) in populations, districts, or countries.

Ecological studies are commonly conducted using data that have already been collected and are available from reliable sources. The investigator may collect and analyze data from districts (or communities or countries) as a whole to determine associations among various factors present in these districts. For instance, a study in the United States collected information on firearm ownership and firearm deaths in various states and analyzed the data. The study found an association between household firearm ownership and firearm death rates during the period 2007–2010 [17]. In this study, the unit of observation was a state and not an individual.

Ecological studies can be used to generate hypotheses about the association between exposure and disease, but they cannot confirm causation. This is because, in ecological studies, it is not clear whether individuals who had the disease had higher exposure than individuals who did not have the disease. The main features of ecological studies are:

- They usually compare mortality or disease prevalence (or incidence) in different groups of people, communities, districts, or countries;
- The unit of observation is the entire community (district, province, or country);
- The estimated exposure level found in that community or geographical unit is a surrogate measure for the exposure of all individuals in that unit;

- Linkage between exposure and outcome (disease or death) at the individual level cannot be ascertained; and
- Ecological studies help in generating hypotheses about the association between exposure and outcome (disease or death), but these studies cannot confirm causation.

5.2.2.1 Types of Ecological Studies

There are three types of ecological studies [18]. They are: a) cross-sectional ecological studies; b) time-trend ecological studies; and c) solely descriptive ecological studies.

In cross-sectional ecological studies, aggregated data on exposure and outcome across communities are compared during the same time period. For example, an investigation might compare the current mortality rate from heart disease across districts with the average cigarette sales in those districts.

Time-trend ecological studies compare variations in aggregated exposures and outcomes over time within the same community (or country or district). For example, a study might investigate whether hospital admissions for asthma in Dhaka city increase on days with higher levels of environmental pollution, such as carbon monoxide in the air.

Solely descriptive ecological studies examine differences in disease incidence or risk factors among communities at a given time or within the same community over time. This study design is used to explore variations in disease incidence (e.g., dengue or oral cancer), mortality rates across districts, or the secular trend of deaths due to cancer or other diseases over a specified period of time in a country.

5.2.2.2 Data Analysis of Ecological Studies

The first step in analyzing ecological study data is to construct a scatter diagram plotting morbidity (or mortality) rates against average exposure rates in each community (or country or geographical area) to assess potential associations between exposure and the outcome of interest. Other measures of association, such as the correlation coefficient (r)[1], coefficient of determination (r^2), and regression coefficient, are also calculated to quantify the relationship between the variables of interest and the outcome [2].

Example

For an ecological study, data on delivery by skilled birth attendants (SBAs) and neonatal mortality rates (NMR) were obtained from a published report for 64 districts in Bangladesh [19]. The objective of the study was to determine the association between delivery by SBAs and NMR. A scatter diagram of NMR against delivery by SBAs was constructed (Figure 5.7), and to quantify the relationship, r (-0.439; p<0.001) and r^2 (0.193) values and regression coefficient (-0.23; p<0.001) were calculated.

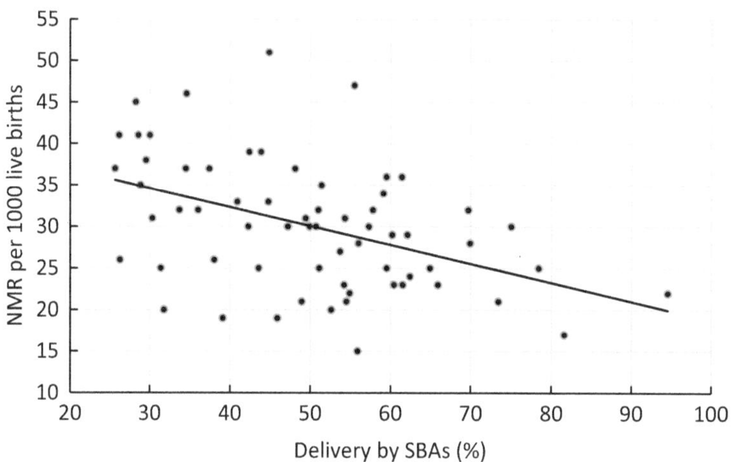

FIGURE 5.7

Scatter diagram of neonatal mortality rates (NMR) and delivery by skilled birth attendants (SBAs). (Drawn with the data from the National Institute of Population Research and Training (NIPORT), International Centre for Diarrhoeal Disease Research, Bangladesh (icddr,b), and MEASURE Evaluation. *Bangladesh District Level Socio-demographic and Health Care Utilization Indicators.* Dhaka, Bangladesh, and Chapel Hill, NC, USA: NIPORT, icddr,b, and MEASURE Evaluation; 2019.)

The scatter diagram shows that there is an inverse linear relationship between delivery by SBAs and NMR (Figure 5.7). An r value of −0.439 (calculated from the data) indicates that there is a significant (p<0.001) negative correlation between delivery by SBAs and NMR, i.e., as the proportion of delivery by SBAs increases, there is a reduction in NMR. On the other hand, the r^2 value of 0.193 indicates that 19.3% of the variation in NMR can be explained by the proportion of delivery by SBAs.

A simple linear regression of NMR on delivery by SBAs was also performed to examine the strength of the association, which is measured by the regression coefficient, or beta (β). The data showed that the regression coefficient was -0.23, indicating that for every 10% increase in delivery by SBAs, NMR decreases by 2.3 per 1,000 live births (p < 0.001).

Though we cannot confirm the association (because the data are not from the individual level), we can propose the hypothesis that "delivery by SBAs prevents neonatal deaths." There are several studies that have confirmed the benefits of delivery by SBAs for the reduction of neonatal deaths [20–22].

Ecological studies, in particular, help in generating hypotheses about the association between exposure and disease. The advantages of such studies are that they utilize the available data from different sources for analysis and can, therefore, be conducted with minimal time and resources. However, the major limitations of such studies are:

- Ecological studies are unable to establish a linkage between exposure and disease among individuals;

- Such studies present the average values of exposure rather than the actual exposure at individual levels; and

- Ecological studies are subjected to potential confounding bias, which cannot be controlled during analysis. For example, suppose that a correlational study found an association between low uptake of antenatal care (ANC) and neonatal mortality. Low uptake of ANC may be a marker (associated with) for a number of other factors, such as a low socio-economic status, low intake of nutrition, including the iron-folic acid tablets, a lack of awareness about immediate newborn care, or other factors. It is not possible to adjust the effects of potential confounding factors while analyzing the data.

Ecological fallacy: When analyzing group-level data for a study, it is important to be aware of the ecological fallacy. The ecological fallacy results from concluding that since an association exists between exposure and disease at the group level, it therefore exists at the individual level [18]. We cannot really conclude this, as we do not know the linkage between exposure and disease at the individual level within the group.

Note

1 The correlation coefficient (r) indicates the degree/strength of the linear relationship between two continuous variables. The value of "r" lies between -1 and $+1$. Values near "zero" indicate no correlation, while values near "plus or minus 1" indicate a strong correlation. A negative value indicates an inverse relationship. A value of $r \geq 0.8$ indicates very strong association; an r value of 0.6 to 0.8 indicates moderately strong association; an r value of 0.3 to 0.5 indicates fair association; and an r value of <0.3 indicates poor association.

   Squaring the "r" value, we get the value for "coefficient of determination (r^2)", which tells us the amount of variation in "Y" due to "X" that can be explained by the regression line. For example, if the r^2 value is 0.7, it indicates that (if Y is body weight and X is height) 70% of the body weight of the individuals can be explained by their height, and the remaining 30% could probably be explained by other factors.

   On the other hand, the *strength of association* between two continuous variables is measured by the regression coefficient (β). The regression coefficient indicates the average increase (or decrease) in Y-value (dependent variable) for each unit variation in X-value (independent variable). For details, students can read any standard biostatistics book.

References

1.   Aggarwal R, Ranganathan P. Study designs: Part 2 – Descriptive studies. *Perspect Clin Res.* 2019;10(1):34–6.

2.   Hennekens CH, Buring JE. *Epidemiology in Medicine.* Boston/Toronto: Little Brown and Company; 1987.

3.   Gordis L. *Epidemiology.* 5th ed. Philadelphia: Elsevier Saunders; 2014.

4.   Centers for Disease Control and Prevention (CDC). *Lesson 1: Introduction to Epidemiology; Section 6: Descriptive Epidemiology;* 2012. Available from: https://archive.cdc.gov/www_cdc_gov/csels/dsepd/ss1978/lesson1/section6.html

5.   Bonita R, Beaglehole R, Kjellström T. *Basic Epidemiology.* 2nd ed. Geneva: World Health Organization; 2006.

6.   Supanvanich S, Podhipak A. *Principles of Epidemiology.* Bangkok: Mahidol University; 1991.

7.   Omair A. Selecting the appropriate study design for your research: Descriptive study designs. *J Health Spec.* 2015;3(3):153–6.

8.   Haque U, Overgaard HJ, Clements ACA, Norris DE, Islam N, Karim J, et al. Malaria burden and control in Bangladesh and prospects for elimination: An epidemiological and economic assessment. *Lancet Glob Health.* 2014;2(2):e98–105. doi:10.1016/S2214-109X(13)70176-1

9.   Naylor GM, Gotoda T, Dixon M, Shimoda T, Gatta L, Owen R, et al. Why does Japan have a high incidence of gastric cancer? Comparison of gastritis between UK and Japanese patients. *Gut.* 2006;55(11):1545–52. doi:10.1136/gut.2005.080358

10. Ghavamzadeh A, Moussavi A, Jahani M, Rastegarpanah M, Iravani M. Esophageal cancer in Iran. *Semin Oncol.* 2001;28(2):153–7. doi:10.1016/s0093-7754(01)90086-7

11. Mutsuddy P, Jhora ST, Shamsuzzaman AKM, Kaisar SM , Khan MNA, Dhiman S, et al. Dengue situation in Bangladesh: An epidemiological shift in terms of morbidity and mortality. *Can J Infect Dis Med Microbiol.* 2019;2019:3516284. doi:10.1155/2019/3516284

12. National Institute of Population Research and Training (NIPORT), International Centre for Diarrhoeal Disease Research, Bangladesh (icddr,b), and MEASURE Evaluation. *Bangladesh Maternal Mortality and Health Care Survey 2016: Final Report.* Dhaka, Bangladesh, and Chapel Hill, NC, USA: NIPORT, icddr,b, and MEASURE Evaluation; 2019.

13. Gottlieb GJ, Ragaz A, Vogel JV, Friedman-Kien A, Rywlin AM, Weiner EA, et al. A preliminary communication on extensively disseminated Kaposi's sarcoma in young homosexual men. *Am J Dermatopathol.* 1981;3(2):111–4.

14. Phupong V. Dengue fever in pregnancy: A case report. *BMC Pregnancy Childbirth.* 2001;1:7. Available from: www.biomedcentral.com/1471-2393/1/7

15. Araújo SA, Moreira DR, Veloso JMR, Neves SP, Pereira RMD, Ribeiro LFC, et al. Fatal staphylococcal infection following classic dengue fever. *Am J Trop Med Hyg.* 2010;83(3):679–82. doi:10.4269/ajtmh.2010.10-0009

16. Carter E, Chandarana P, Duggineni S, Grewal R, Kheraj A, Saleh W. Case series of extra pulmonary tuberculosis presenting as facial swelling. *Br Dent J.* 2015;218(9):519–22. doi:10.1038/sj.bdj.2015.342

17. Fleegler EW, Lee LK, Monuteaux MC, Hemenway D, Mannix R. Firearm legislation and firearm-related fatalities in the United States. *JAMA Intern Med.* 2013;173(9):732–40. doi:10.1001/jamainternmed.2013.1286

18. Ibrahim M, Alexander L, Shy C, Farr S. Ecologic studies. *UNC School of Public Health: ERIC Notebook.* 2000;12:1–3. Available from: https://sph.unc.edu/wp-content/uploads/sites/112/2015/07/nciph_ERIC9.pdf

19. National Institute of Population Research and Training (NIPORT), International Centre for Diarrhoeal Disease Research, Bangladesh (icddr,b), and MEASURE Evaluation. *Bangladesh District Level Socio-demographic and Health Care Utilization Indicators.* Dhaka, Bangladesh, and Chapel Hill, NC, USA: NIPORT, icddr,b, and MEASURE Evaluation; 2019.

20. Baruwa OJ, Amoateng AY , Mkwananzi S. Association between type of birth attendants and neonatal mortality: Evidence from a national survey. *Afr Health Sci.* 2021;21(4):1870–6. doi:10.4314/ahs.v21i4.45

21. Singh K, Brodish P, Suchindran C. A regional multilevel analysis: Can skilled birth attendants uniformly decrease neonatal mortality? *Matern Child Health J.* 2014;18(1):242–9. doi:10.1007/s10995-013-1260-7

22. Titaley CR, Dibley MJ, Agho K, Roberts CL, Hall J. Determinants of neonatal mortality in Indonesia. *BMC Public Health.* 2008;8:232. doi:10.1186/1471-2458-8-232

6

Cross-Sectional Studies

Mohammad Tajul Islam

Cross-sectional studies are a type of observational study design. Cross-sectional studies are also called prevalence surveys. The main objectives of cross-sectional studies are to describe the patterns of disease prevalence (not incidence) in the community (or population) at a certain point in time and to test the association between possible risk factors and disease for the development of research questions and formulation of hypotheses. In cross-sectional studies, individuals are not followed forward. The exposure and outcome among individuals are measured at the same time. Therefore, cross-sectional studies provide a "snapshot" of the diseased and non-diseased individuals in the population [1–6].

Since the exposure and outcome are measured at the same time, in many instances, it is not possible to determine whether the exposure preceded or resulted from the disease (temporal relationship). For example, a cross-sectional study found an association between undernutrition and persistent diarrhea (diarrhea lasting for more than 14 days) among children. It is very difficult to say from the cross-sectional data whether undernutrition is responsible for persistent diarrhea or whether undernutrition is a consequence of persistent diarrhea. Such a dilemma is virtually common in all cross-sectional studies.

In cross-sectional studies, prevalence is affected by the outmigration of diseased individuals from the study area. For example, workers affected by the factory environment (e.g., in an asbestos factory) may quit their jobs and migrate to other factories or areas.

Cross-sectional studies reflect the current health status of a community. Such a study is valuable both to public health administrators and epidemiologists. Health administrators use the cross-sectional study findings to understand the health status of the community, the extent and distribution of health problems, priority setting, efficient allocation of resources, and intervention planning, whereas epidemiologists use the data to identify potential risk factors, design analytical studies to confirm them, and

DOI: 10.1201/9781003654803-6

provide recommendations for preventive interventions [1, 2, 4]. For example, in Bangladesh, the Demographic and Health Survey (DHS) is conducted every three years, collecting information through household interviews from a random sample of the population. It provides valuable information on fertility, mortality, nutritional status, child health, and maternal health for effective health care planning and administration. Cross-sectional studies can also be conducted to study occupational exposure and the prevalence of diseases in relation to that exposure.

6.1 Types of Cross-Sectional Studies

Cross-sectional studies are of two types: *descriptive cross-sectional studies and analytic cross-sectional studies*. In descriptive cross-sectional studies, the prevalence of a disease is measured at a particular point in time (point prevalence) or over a specified period of time (period prevalence) in the specified population. In descriptive cross-sectional studies, the prevalence of a disease between exposed and unexposed subjects is not statistically compared.

On the other hand, in analytic cross-sectional studies, data on the prevalence of disease and exposure are cross-classified for the purpose of comparison. The differences in disease prevalence between exposed and unexposed groups are then statistically analyzed to find an association. This type of analysis helps researchers to evaluate risk factors and develop hypotheses about the relationship between exposure and outcome. The basic difference between descriptive and analytic cross-sectional studies is that in analytic cross-sectional studies, hypotheses are tested, whereas hypotheses are not tested in descriptive cross-sectional studies.

6.2 Conduct

Cross-sectional studies are usually conducted by taking a representative sample from a defined population of interest. If the population size is small, the whole population may be studied, provided there are enough resources available for this. To have a representative sample from the population, the sample may be drawn through either of the following methods: a) simple random sampling; b) systematic random sampling; c) stratified random sampling; or d) cluster sampling (see Chapter 18). Once the sample is drawn, information on exposures and outcomes is collected from the study participants through questionnaire interviews, observations, physical examinations, and/or laboratory examinations.

6.3 Data Analysis

From the data of a cross-sectional study, we can calculate the prevalence of a disease in the community and the factors associated with it. Data are commonly analyzed using descriptive statistics (such as frequency, percentage, mean, median, standard deviation, and quartiles) and presented in the form of tables, graphs, or charts (descriptive cross-sectional studies).

To identify the factors associated with a disease (analytic cross-sectional studies), cross-tabulations of data on exposure(s) and disease are done, and relevant analytic statistical methods (e.g., chi-square test or others) are used. In addition, two types of measures of association can be calculated from cross-sectional data to quantify the relationship. They are the *prevalence ratio* and the *prevalence odds ratio* [7].

The prevalence ratio (PR) is analogous to the relative risk (RR) that we calculate in cohort studies. The prevalence ratio is the ratio of the disease prevalence among the exposed group to the disease prevalence among the unexposed group. It compares the prevalence of disease in individuals who are exposed to the prevalence of disease in those who are unexposed. The prevalence ratio is calculated when the outcome occurs over a short period of time. For example, one could calculate the prevalence ratio for an acute outbreak of a disease, such as measles, dengue, or tuberculosis.

On the other hand, the prevalence odds ratio (POR) is the preferred measure of association in studies of chronic diseases (e.g., asthma, diabetes mellitus, or hypertension) or the association of long-lasting risk factors (e.g., smoking, exposure to arsenic, or high serum cholesterol level) with diseases, such as heart disease or cancer [8–10]. The prevalence odds ratio is the ratio of the odds of disease in the exposed group to the odds of disease in the unexposed group. The prevalence odds ratio is calculated in the same manner as we calculate the odds ratio (OR) in case-control studies (see Chapter 7). The prevalence ratio and the prevalence odds ratio will be similar if the disease prevalence in both exposed and unexposed groups is low (below 10%).

Cross-sectional studies are particularly useful to study chronic diseases where the onset of the disease is difficult to determine (e.g., rheumatoid arthritis, diabetes, asthma, and hypertension) or for long-lasting risk factors such as smoking, hypercholesterolemia, and arsenicosis. Therefore, the prevalence odds ratio is commonly used as a measure of association in cross-sectional studies [6, 9, 10].

Example

A cross-sectional study was conducted in a district with the objectives of determining the prevalence of self-reported diabetes mellitus and examining its association with sex. To conduct the study, a random sample of 460 individuals aged over 30 years was drawn from the study population, and relevant data were collected. Among the 460 participants selected for the study, 50 reported that they had diabetes. Data from the study subjects are cross-tabulated by diabetes status and sex and are presented in Table 6.1.

One of the study objectives was to determine if there is an association between sex and diabetes. Therefore, the null hypothesis is "there is no association between sex and diabetes in the population" and the alternative hypothesis is "there is an association between sex and diabetes in the population".

From the data, we can calculate the overall prevalence of diabetes in the population as well as the prevalence among males and females (to address the first objective). The prevalence of a disease is the proportion of individuals who have the disease in a population. The prevalence of diabetes (in our example) can be calculated using the following formula:

$$\text{Prevalence of diabetes in the population} = \frac{\text{No. reported to have diabetes}}{\text{Total no. of people surveyed}}$$

Or,

$$\text{Prevalence (overall) of diabetes in the population} = \frac{50}{460} \times 100 = 10.9\%$$

We can also calculate the prevalence of diabetes among males and females as follows:

$$\text{Prevalence of diabetes in females} = \frac{\text{No. of females who have diabetes}}{\text{Total no. of females surveyed}}$$

Or,

TABLE 6.1

Frequency distribution of diabetes by sex

| | Diabetes | | |
	Present	Absent	Total
Female	32 (a)	208 (b)	240 (a + b)
Male	18 (c)	202 (d)	220 (c + d)
Total	50 (a + c)	410 (b + d)	460 (n)

$$\text{Prevalence of diabetes in females} = \frac{32}{240} \times 100 = 13.3\%$$

Similarly,

$$\text{Prevalence of diabetes in males} = \frac{18}{220} \times 100 = 8.2\%$$

Data show that the overall prevalence of diabetes in the population is 10.9%. Data also indicate that the prevalence of diabetes is higher among females (13.3%) than males (8.2%).

To find whether there is an association between sex and diabetes, we will use the chi-square (χ^2) test. The chi-square test is an appropriate method to find an association between two categorical variables, such as sex and diabetes [11]. The formula for the chi-square test (using symbols of Table 6.1) is (appropriate only for a two by two table):

$$\text{Chi-square, } \chi^2 = \frac{n(ad - bc)^2}{(a+b)(c+d)(a+c)(b+d)}$$

$$\text{Chi-square, } \chi^2 = \frac{460 \times (32 \times 202 - 18 \times 208)^2}{(240 \times 220 \times 410 \times 50)} = 3.14$$

In this example, the χ^2 calculated value is 3.14, which is less than the tabulated value of 3.841 [obtained from the chi-square distribution table at 5% level of significance and one degree of freedom (df)] with a degree of freedom (df) of one (for a two by two table, the degree of freedom is one) [11]. The p-value for the test is 0.076 (obtained by SPSS; you can also find it from the chi-square table). Since the p-value is greater than 0.05, we cannot reject the null hypothesis at a 95% confidence level. This indicates that, though there is a difference in the prevalence of diabetes among males and females in the sample, there may not be any significant difference in the prevalence among males and females in the population. In the same manner, associations between other factors of interest and diabetes can be determined.

Since we cannot calculate the incidence of diabetes among females and males from the cross-sectional data, we cannot calculate the relative risk (RR), which is a direct measure of risk (see Chapter 8) for the causation of a disease. Instead, we can calculate either the PR or POR to quantify the association, as discussed earlier. Since diabetes is a chronic condition, it is preferable to calculate the POR. However, for the purpose of discussion, we will calculate both PR and POR. The PR of diabetes (female to male) is given by:

$$\text{Prevalence ratio, PR} = \frac{\text{Prevalence of diabetes in females}}{\text{Prevalence of diabetes in males}}$$

Or,

$$\text{Prevalence ratio, PR} = \frac{13.3}{8.2} = 1.62$$

We can also calculate the POR as follows (see Chapter 7):

$$\text{Prevalence odds ratio, POR} = \frac{ad}{bc}$$

Or,

$$\text{Prevalence odds ratio, POR} = \frac{32 \times 202}{208 \times 18} = 1.73$$

In our example, the PR is 1.62. A PR of 1.62 indicates that the prevalence of diabetes is 1.62 times (or 62%) higher among females than males. On the other hand, a POR of 1.73 indicates that females are 1.73 times more likely to have diabetes compared to males (or, the odds of diabetes are 1.73 times higher among females than males). It is necessary to calculate the confidence intervals to further interpret the PR and POR. For more details, refer to Chapters 7 and 8.

There are numerous published articles on cross-sectional studies in journals. Though some references [8–10] are provided in this chapter, readers may go through some other publications to get more information about the design and analysis of cross-sectional studies.

6.4 Advantages and Limitations

The advantages and limitations of cross-sectional studies are discussed in Chapter 4. In short, the main advantages are that such studies can be conducted with limited time and resources and help researchers in generating hypotheses. The main limitations of such studies are that, commonly, the temporal relationship may not be established, and the prevalence of disease is affected due to the outmigration of diseased individuals.

6.5 Potential Biases in Cross-Sectional Studies

Cross-sectional studies are subject to two broad types of bias. They are: a) selection bias and b) information bias. One type of selection bias that may occur in cross-sectional studies is *sampling bias*. Sampling bias arises from a faulty sampling frame and/or faulty selection of study subjects from the study population. On the other hand, information bias may occur in cross-sectional studies due to the case definition used for the detection of cases. This is due to the inherent characteristics of the case definition (or a diagnostic test), such as its sensitivity and specificity, which may result in the misclassification of diseased and non-diseased individuals (see Chapters 7 and 11).

Other types of bias that may affect a cross-sectional study include incidence-prevalence bias and temporal bias. The incidence-prevalence bias is a kind of selection bias, while the temporal bias is a kind of information bias. All these forms of bias should be carefully considered when designing a cross-sectional study and interpreting its results.

6.5.1 Incidence-Prevalence Bias

Incidence-prevalence bias may result when prevalence data (cross-sectional data) are used to estimate the relative risk. In cross-sectional studies, sometimes the strength of the association between exposure and outcome is measured in terms of the prevalence ratio. If the investigator is interested in evaluating the causal association, the use of the prevalence ratio (PR) as an estimate of the relative risk (RR) is subject to bias. It can be shown that the odds of prevalence are equal to the product of the incidence and duration of the disease [7]. That is:

$$\text{Prevalence odds} = \frac{\text{Prevalence}}{(1 - \text{Prevalence})} = \text{Incidence} \times \text{Duration}$$

Or,

$$\text{Prevalence} = \text{Incidence} \times \text{Duration} \times (1 - \text{Prevalence})$$

We know that the prevalence ratio (PR) is calculated as:

$$PR = \frac{\text{Prevalece of disease among exposed}}{\text{Prevalence of disease among unexposed}}$$

Therefore,

$$PR = \frac{\text{Incidence} \times \text{Duration} \times (1 - \text{Prevalence}) \left[\text{in exposed}\right]}{\text{Incidence} \times \text{Duration} \times (1 - \text{Prevalence}) \left[\text{in unexposed}\right]}$$

Or,

$$PR = RR \times \frac{\text{Duration}(\text{in exposed})}{\text{Duration}(\text{in unexposed})} \times \frac{(1-\text{Prevalence})[\text{in exposed}]}{(1-\text{Prevalence})[\text{in unexposed}]}$$

The equation above shows that the PR is not equal to the RR but is a function of three factors. They are: factor "A (the relative risk or RR)", factor "B (the ratio of disease duration among exposed and unexposed)", and factor "C [the ratio of the term (1 – Prevalence) among exposed and unexposed]".

The factors "B" (the ratio of disease duration among exposed and unexposed) and "C" [the ratio of the term (1 – Prevalence) among exposed and unexposed] represent two types of biases. They are called the *duration ratio bias or survival bias* and the *point prevalence complement ratio bias*, respectively.

If exposure affects the disease's survival time (for example, if the survival time of a disease is shorter among the exposed compared to the unexposed), the estimate will be subjected to survival bias. However, if the duration of survival of a disease among exposed and unexposed groups is the same and the prevalence of disease is low (less than 10%) among exposed and unexposed groups, the PR will be a good estimate of the RR. More details about the biases in cross-sectional studies can be found elsewhere [7].

6.5.2 Temporal Bias

In cross-sectional studies, the temporal sequence of exposure and outcome (whether exposure occurred before or after the outcome) needs to be confirmed before establishing a causal association. In many instances, it is difficult to firmly establish the temporal relationship (except for fixed factors such as gender, blood group, and genetic codes) in cross-sectional studies.

References

1. Hennekens CH, Buring JE. *Epidemiology in Medicine*. Boston/Toronto: Little Brown and Company; 1987.
2. Gordis L. *Epidemiology*. 5th ed. Philadelphia: Elsevier Saunders; 2014.
3. Lilienfeld DE, Stolley PD. *Foundations of Epidemiology*. 3rd ed. New York: Oxford University Press; 1994.
4. Supanvanich S, Podhipak A. *Principles of Epidemiology*. Bangkok: Mahidol University; 1991.
5. Ibrahim M, Alexander L, Shy C. Cross-sectional studies. *UNC School of Public Health: ERIC Notebook*. 1999;7:1–4.
6. Setia MS. Methodology Series Module 3: Cross-sectional Studies. *Indian J Dermatol*. 2016;61(3):261–4. doi:10.4103/0019-5154.182410

7.   Szklo M, Nieto FJ. *Epidemiology: Beyond the Basics.* 2nd ed. Boston: Jones and Bartlett Publishers; 2007.

8.   Zhang H, Ni J, Yu C, et al. Sex-based differences in diabetes prevalence and risk factors: A population-based cross-sectional study among low-income adults in China. *Front Endocrinol.* 2019;10:658. doi:10.3389/fendo.2019.00658

9.   Liu X, Zhang L, Zhang F, et al. Prevalence and risk factors of active tuberculosis in patients with rheumatic diseases: A multi-center, cross-sectional study in China. *Emerg Microbes Infect.* 2021;10(1):2303–12. doi:10.1080/22221751.2021.2004864

10. Yang H, Haldeman S, Lu ML, et al. Low back pain prevalence and related workplace psychosocial risk factors: A study using data from the 2010 National Health Interview Survey. *J Manipulative Physiol Ther.* 2016;39(7):459–72. doi:10.1016/j.jmpt.2016.07.004

11. Daniel WW. *Biostatistics: A Foundation for Analysis in the Health Sciences.* 7th ed. New York: Wiley; 1999.

7
Case-Control Studies

Mohammad Tajul Islam

Case-control studies are important observational analytic study designs in epidemiology to determine the factors that cause or prevent disease. The main objective of case-control studies is to find associations between exposure (to one or more factors) and outcome (disease). The term "association", used in connection with exposure to a factor and a disease, indicates that the factor is either linked with an increase or decrease in risk for the development of the disease. In a case-control design, "cases" are individuals with the disease under study, and "controls" are similar individuals without the disease. Information is collected from both cases and controls on past and existing exposure to factors that are thought to be associated with the disease of interest. The investigator then compares the rates of exposure in both groups to find an association [1–5].

Case-control studies are popularly known as "retrospective studies". The basic difference between case-control and cohort studies is that case-control studies begin with the outcome (disease), while cohort studies begin with the exposure.

7.1 Design

To examine the possible association between exposure and disease, a group of people is selected who have the disease (cases), and for the purpose of comparison, another group of people is identified who do not have the disease (controls). The proportion of people exposed to the factor of interest in the past is then ascertained in both cases and controls. If the exposure is associated with an increased risk of disease, it is anticipated that the proportion of cases exposed will be higher than the proportion of controls exposed. Because of the design, it is not possible to calculate the incidence

DOI: 10.1201/9781003654803-7

and prevalence rates of a disease from the data of a case-control study [1, 6]. The main features of case-control studies are:

- The relevant outcome has already occurred by the time the study begins;
- The study involves a group of people with the disease of interest and an appropriate control group;
- This design is an indirect approach to measuring the risk (in terms of the odds ratio) of a disease for a specific exposure;
- The incidence and prevalence rates of a disease cannot be calculated from the data; and
- Relative risk (RR) cannot be measured directly from this design, but the odds ratio (OR) calculated in a case-control study is an estimate of the RR.

7.2 Types of Case-Control Studies

The case-control studies are primarily of two types. They are: a) unmatched case-control studies; and b) matched case-control studies. In unmatched case-control studies, controls are selected without matching with cases, while in matched case-control studies, controls are matched with one or more characteristics (e.g., age, gender, ethnicity, hypertension, or others) with cases [1, 2]. Case-control studies can also be classified as follows based on the way the cases and controls are selected for the study [7].

7.2.1 Case-Based Case-Control Study

This is the most commonly used design and is the simplest strategy to select cases and controls for a case-control study. Here, cases and controls are identified and selected from the same reference population. For example, a case-control study, where incidence cases (new cases) are selected from a hospital, and controls are also selected from the same hospital during the same time period.

7.2.2 Case-Control Studies Within a Cohort Study

Case-control studies can be designed within an ongoing cohort study. In a well-defined cohort study, both cases and controls can be selected, and data are analyzed to identify the factors associated with the outcome (disease). Case-control studies conducted within a defined cohort study are also called *hybrid designs*.

In a cohort study, if controls are selected at the beginning from the base population of the cohort and cases are selected from the same cohort that occur during the specified follow-up period, it is called a *case-cohort* study. After selecting the cases and controls from the cohort, they are compared for exposure to certain factors to find associations. The advantage of taking controls from the base population is that the same control group can be used to investigate different outcomes (diseases) within the cohort study.

Another design, where cases and controls are selected from within a defined cohort study, is the *nested case-control* study. In this design, controls are not selected at the beginning from the base population. Rather, controls are randomly selected from individuals at risk (within the cohort) whenever there is an occurrence of a case (disease) during the follow-up period. Such a sampling strategy for selecting the control group is called the *incidence density sampling or risk-set sampling*. Incidence density sampling is equivalent to matching cases and controls on the duration of follow-up and permits the use of standard statistical techniques for data analysis.

Case-control studies within a cohort study (case-cohort or nested case-control study) are primarily used to reduce cost. For example, a researcher interested in evaluating the effect of vitamin D deficiency on the development of colon cancer may use a hybrid study design. At the beginning of the cohort study, blood samples from all subjects can be collected and preserved. During the follow-up period, cancer cases are identified within the cohort. Once a sufficient number of cases is available for a case-control study, cases are compared with controls selected either at the base (case-cohort study) or concurrently with the occurrence of each case (nested case-control study). The blood samples of only the cases and controls are then analyzed for vitamin D levels. With this design, the risk factor can be evaluated at a much lower cost, as fewer blood samples need to be analyzed. Such a design also ensures the presence of exposure before the outcome.

7.3 Definition of Cases and Controls

The first step in designing a case-control study is to define the case or disease of interest. The case definition is a set of standard criteria for deciding whether an individual would be classified as having the disease of interest. Strict diagnostic criteria (preferably the gold standard) for diseases need to be considered when conducting a case-control study. The case definition should include the clinical criteria, which should be clear and objective. The criteria for defining a case should be set in such a way that they represent a disease as homogeneously as possible, as similar manifestations can often be found in different diseases with varying etiologies. For example, cervical cancer and uterine cancer may present with similar clinical manifestations, but their risk factors are different. The risk factors for uterine cancer are a low number of sexual partners and a high socio-economic status, while the risk factors for cervical cancer are a high number of sexual partners, a low socio-economic status, and human papillomavirus infection.

Similar to cases, controls should also be clearly defined. For example, Fukai et al. (2021) conducted a case-control study to investigate the risks of cardio-vascular diseases (CVD) associated with specific occupations [8]. In this study, the authors defined cases (CVD) as "patients with a diagnosis at admission of cerebral infarction, intracerebral hemorrhage, subarachnoid hemorrhage, or acute myocardial infarction" and controls as "patients who were admitted at the same hospital and during the same period for reasons other than diseases of the circulatory system". Other examples of case-control studies can be found elsewhere [9–11].

7.4 Selection of Cases and Controls

Once the case definition is fixed, cases can be selected from a number of sources, such as hospitals, the general population, or the community, at a single point in time or over a specified period of time. If cases are selected from one or more hospitals, it is called a *hospital-based case-control study*, and when cases are selected from the population, it is called a *population-based case-control study*.

The specific advantage of population-based case-control studies is that they avoid selection bias arising from hospitalization. However, due to the high costs associated with population-based case-control studies, they are not commonly conducted.

Cases for a case-control study can be selected in different ways. The cases can be selected from:

a) Prevalence cases (existing cases): If the disease is rare, the inclusion of prevalence cases (over a specific time period) will make it easier to find the cases for the study;

b) Incidence cases (newly diagnosed cases): It is always preferable to select newly diagnosed cases over a specified period of time.

Inclusion of prevalence cases is suitable when the disease incidence is very low. The selection of prevalence cases saves time and money. However, there can be problems with the interpretation of the results. Prevalent cases are usually the ones that survive the acute condition. Therefore, prevalent cases may indicate the determinants of survival in addition to risk factors for the disease. Moreover, the inclusion of prevalent cases is more susceptible to recall bias compared to incident cases. Temporal sequences can be more clearly established if incidence cases are selected, compared to prevalence cases. Therefore, whenever possible, it is preferable to consider the incidence cases for a case-control study.

The selection of an appropriate control group is perhaps the most difficult issue in a case-control design. Controls are individuals who do not have the disease under investigation. The general principle is that controls should be comparable to cases as regards to all factors except for the exposure of interest.

Sometimes it is necessary to exclude certain study subjects. If any exclusion criteria are set for the selection of cases, the same exclusion criteria should be applied for the selection of controls. Controls should be selected from patients who presented with similar symptoms to those of the cases but were diagnosed as not having the disease. Controls should be selected from the same population from which cases are selected, i.e., controls should be representative of the population from which cases are selected. Such a case-control study will then provide a valid estimation of the association between exposure and disease.

In like cases, hospital patients are the most common source of controls, such as individuals seeking medical care at the same hospital for conditions other than the disease of interest. Controls can also be selected from the community (i.e., a random sample from the general population from which the cases are selected), friends, neighbors, or relatives. The advantages of selecting controls from hospitals are:

- Controls are readily available, cost-effective, and take less time to select;

- Cases and controls equally remember the past events of exposure and thus, minimize the recall bias;

- Hospital patients are more cooperative; and

- Patients are coming to the hospital from similar socio-economic and cultural backgrounds.

The main disadvantage of the hospital controls is that the group may differ from healthy individuals in terms of exposure. On the other hand, the disadvantages of selecting community controls are unavailability, nonresponse, and costly data collection.

To enable the investigator to determine the true effect of exposure on an outcome, cases and controls should be selected from the same population group.

TABLE 7.1

Guidelines for sources of cases and controls in case-control studies

Cases	Controls
All cases diagnosed in a single hospital	Sample of patients in same hospital where cases were selected
All cases diagnosed in one or more hospitals	Sample of individuals who are residents in same block or neighborhood of cases
All cases diagnosed in all hospitals in the community	Controls should be from sample of patients in all hospitals in the community without the disease of interest
All cases diagnosed in a sample of the general population	Controls should be a random sample of the general population
All cases diagnosed in the community (hospitals, doctors' clinic, or other medical facilities)	Controls should be a random sample of the general population of that community
Cases selected by any of the above methods	Spouses, siblings, or associates (schoolmates or workmates) of cases

A guideline for the selection of controls for each type of case is provided in Table 7.1 [4].

7.5 Number of Control Groups and Number of Controls per Case

Ideally, a case-control study should have a single control group. However, multiple control groups may be necessary under certain circumstances. For instance, to examine the association between coffee consumption and pancreatic cancer in a hospital-based case-control study, if it is anticipated that hospital controls may differ from the general population in terms of coffee consumption, it is preferable to consider two control groups—one from the hospital where cases are selected and another from the community. Consistency of results among studies where different types of control groups are used increases the validity and generalizability of study findings.

Once the source and number of control groups are decided, it is necessary to decide how many controls to select for each case. When the number of cases and controls available is large, a ratio of 1:1 (one control for each case) is optimum. When the number of cases available for the study is limited, the ratio can be changed to 1:2 or 1:3. As the number of controls per case increases, the power of the study also increases. However, it is not rational to have a case-control ratio beyond 1:4 since it does not contribute anymore to the study power.

7.6 Ascertainment of Exposure

Information on past (before development of the disease) and existing exposures of interest needs to be ascertained from both cases and controls for the purpose of analysis. Depending on the nature of the exposure, there are several approaches to obtain information. Data on exposure and confounding factors are commonly obtained from personal recall through an interview or a self-administered questionnaire. When using a questionnaire for data collection through interviews, all cases and controls must be asked the same questions in the same manner. Existing health or clinical records, physical examinations (e.g., blood pressure, body weight, and height), and laboratory tests on sera or tissue from both cases and controls can also be used to collect exposure data. Regardless of the method used, it is important that the ascertainment of exposure status is comparable between cases and controls.

The validity of information obtained from study subjects depends in part on the subjects themselves and the completeness and quality of hospital records. People may be able to remember quite well where they lived or what jobs they did in the past. On the contrary, long-term recall of exposure to a factor or utilization of services (e.g., use of a drug during pregnancy, receiving antenatal care, or birthweight of the baby) is probably less reliable.

7.7 Matched Case-Control Designs

Matching means pairing cases with one or more controls based on their similarities. Cases may be matched with controls with regard to one or more characteristics, such as age, sex, socio-economic condition, blood group, ethnicity, or other factors.

There are two ways to match cases with controls: a) individual matching and b) group matching. Individual matching is usually done during the sampling stage of the study, when controls are selected for cases. Individual matching can also be done during data analysis (post-matching). In this case (post-matching), cases are paired with controls after the unmatched controls have been selected for the study.

Group matching is also possible in a case-control study. In this approach, cases are selected first. The proportion of the factor to be matched is then calculated among cases, and controls are selected based on this proportion. For example, suppose a researcher aims to match cases and controls by gender in a case-control study. To conduct the study, the researcher has selected 150 cases, of which 30% are female. If the case-control ratio is 1:1, the researcher should select 150 controls, ensuring that 30% of them are also female.

The primary objective of matching is to eliminate biased comparisons between cases and controls. However, this objective can only be achieved if the data analysis is in line with the matched design, i.e., the matched design should follow the matched analysis. Another objective of matching is to achieve a balance in the number of cases and controls at each level of the matching variable. For example, if cases and controls are matched based on gender, there will be an equal number of cases and controls for both males and females.

7.7.1 Criteria for Matching

The primary objective of matching is to control extraneous factors (confounding factors) that may influence the exposure-outcome relationship. Matching should, therefore, be done for variables that are associated with the outcome and/or the exposure of interest. Matching cases with controls is appropriate in the following situations (Figure 7.1) [3]:

- When the matching variable is a confounding factor, i.e., when the matching variable is associated with the exposure and causally associated with the disease (i.e., a risk factor for the disease). In this situation, failure to control the matching variable would provide a biased estimate of the effect of exposure on disease.

- When there is an interaction between the matching variable and exposure, and the matching variable is independently associated with the outcome (disease). In this situation, if the matching variable is not controlled, the data may show an indirect association (spurious association) between the exposure and the disease, which is actually due to the interaction between the exposure and the matching variable.

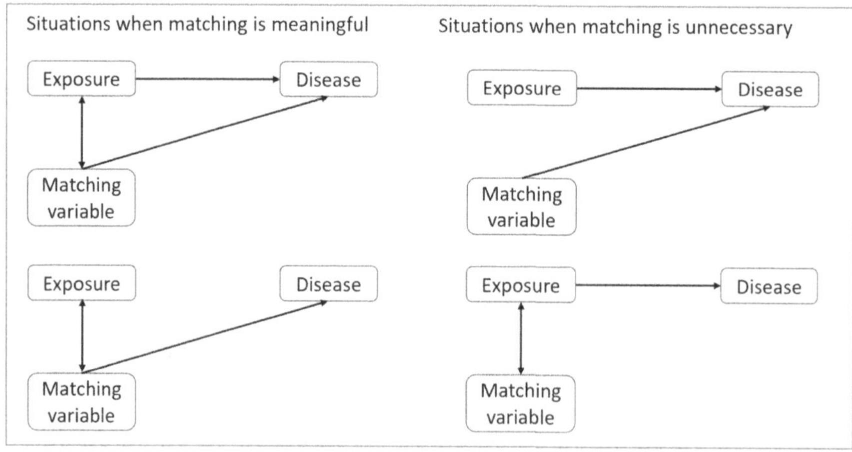

FIGURE 7.1
Situations for matching of cases and controls.

On the other hand, matching for a third variable is unnecessary in the following situations:

- When both the exposure and the matching variable are independently associated with the outcome (disease) without any interaction between them. In this situation, it may seem logical to match for the matching variable since it is associated with the outcome (disease). However, because there is no interaction between the exposure and the matching variable, matching will not alter the association between the exposure and the disease.
- Another situation in which matching is unnecessary is when the matching variable is associated with the exposure but is not an independent risk factor for the disease (i.e., it is not associated with the disease).

7.7.2 Advantages and Disadvantages of Matching

Matched case-control studies have the following advantages:

- Matching makes cases and controls comparable to the factors matched;
- The process of matching achieves a balance between cases and controls;
- Matching eliminates the influence of an extraneous factor (the matching variable) in the relationship between exposure and disease. Therefore, it is not necessary to adjust for the variable matched during analysis;
- A smaller sample size is required to test a hypothesis between exposure and outcome; and
- Matching done on a strong confounder tends to increase the power of the study.

However, there are a number of limitations to matching. They include:

- As controls are matched with cases, it is not possible to assess the risk contributed by the factor(s) matched for the outcome;
- Matching may increase the cost and length of time required to find matches;
- There is a loss of information on unmatched individuals;
- Matching increases the complexity of the control selection process (e.g., you may look for a control who is a female, aged 45–46 years, and has blood group B, but you may not get such a match during the desired time period. Therefore, post-matching is sometimes useful);
- A certain fraction of cases are often discarded due to the lack of a suitable matched control within the time frame;

- Matching sometimes ends up with overmatching; and
- Matching tends to reduce the external validity, though the internal validity is improved.

7.8 Data Analysis of Case-Control Studies

7.8.1 Data Analysis of an Unmatched Case-Control Design

Example

A case-control study is designed to test the hypothesis whether or not maternal malnutrition is a risk factor for low birthweight (LBW; birthweight less than 2,500 gm). To test the hypothesis, 200 new-born babies weighing less than 2,500 gm (cases) were selected from a maternity hospital, and an equal number of normal-weight (weighing ≥2,500 gm) new-born babies (controls) were selected from the same maternity hospital. The nutritional status of mothers was obtained from the antenatal check-up records. The data obtained from the study is presented in Table 7.2.

Data from a case-control study are analyzed to calculate the odds ratio (OR). We cannot calculate the incidence or prevalence of a disease and, thus, the relative risk (RR) in a case-control design. The OR is an indirect measure of risk. The OR of disease and the OR of exposure are mathematically equivalent. Therefore, the OR of exposure to a disease is equivalent to the OR of the disease if the person is exposed.

Odds are the probability of success (e.g., exposed) divided by the probability of failure (e.g., unexposed). The OR is the ratio of two odds, i.e., the ratio of the odds of exposure if the persons have the disease (cases) to the odds of exposure if the persons do not have the disease (controls). Odds are calculated as:

$$\text{Odds of exposure among cases} = \frac{\text{Probability of exposed (success)}}{\text{Probability of unexposed (failure)}}$$

TABLE 7.2

Data from an unmatched case-control study

	Case	Control
Malnourished	95 (a)	50 (b)
Well-nourished	105 (c)	150 (d)
Total	200 (a + c)	200 (b + d)

Therefore (using symbols of Table 7.2),

$$\text{Odds of exposure among cases} = \frac{a \div (a+c)}{c \div (a+c)} = \frac{a}{c}$$

Similarly,

$$\text{Odds of exposure among controls} = \frac{b \div (b+d)}{d \div (b+d)} = \frac{b}{d}$$

Therefore,

$$\text{Odds ratio, OR} = \frac{(a \div c)}{(b \div d)} = \frac{ad}{bc}$$

In our example, the OR is equal to 2.71 [(95 × 150) ÷ (50 × 105)].

It is important to note that the probability and odds are different. We can convert odds into probability by using the following formula:

$$\text{Probability} = \frac{\text{Odds}}{(1 + \text{Odds})}$$

7.8.2 Interpretation of Odds Ratio

An OR greater than 1 indicates that cases are more likely to be exposed compared to controls. In other words, it can also be stated that those who are exposed are more likely to have the outcome compared to those who are not exposed (i.e., exposure is a risk factor for the outcome). If the OR is less than 1, it indicates that cases are less likely to be exposed compared to controls. This is a situation where exposure is associated with a lower risk of the outcome (i.e., exposure provides some level of protection against the development of the outcome or disease). An OR of 1.0 indicates that there is no association between exposure and outcome, i.e., the exposure does not have any influence on the outcome.

In our example, the OR is 2.71. This indicates that malnourished women are 2.71 times more likely to deliver a low birthweight baby compared to well-nourished women. It can also be stated that the odds of delivering a low birthweight baby are 2.7 times higher for mothers who are malnourished compared to mothers who are well-nourished.

To understand whether the calculated OR is statistically significant or not (i.e., by chance or not), we need to calculate the 95% confidence interval (CI) of the OR. The 95% CI of OR can be calculated by using the following formula (other formulas are also available):

$$95\% \text{ CI of OR} = \text{OR} \times e^{\pm(1.96 \times \text{SE of lnOR})}$$

Here, "ln" is the "natural log" or log base e ($\log_e$), "SE" stands for "standard error", and "e" is a constant, the value of which is 2.71828... .. The antilog of "ln" is the exponential of the value, i.e., e^x. You will find all these mathematical functions on a scientific calculator.

To calculate the 95% CI of OR, first we need to calculate the standard error (SE) of lnOR by using the following formula:

$$\text{SE (standard error) of lnOR} = \sqrt{\left(\frac{1}{a} + \frac{1}{b} + \frac{1}{c} + \frac{1}{d}\right)}$$

In our example, the SE of lnOR is

$$\text{SE (standard error) of lnOR} = \sqrt{\left(\frac{1}{95} + \frac{1}{50} + \frac{1}{105} + \frac{1}{150}\right)} = 0.22$$

Therefore, the 95% CI of OR is:

$$95\% \text{ CI of OR} = 2.71 \times e^{\pm(1.96 \times 0.22)}$$

i.e., 95% CI of OR is 1.75 – 4.14 (you can easily calculate it with a scientific calculator).

The interpretation of the 95% CI for the OR is similar to the interpretation of the 95% CI for the relative risk (RR) (see Section 8.5.1). To interpret the 95% CI for the OR, we examine the range of the interval. In this example, the 95% CI is 1.75 – 4.14. If the range of the 95% CI includes one, the OR is not statistically significant, i.e., there is no significant association between exposure and outcome. Since the range of our calculated 95% CI does not include one, there is a significant association between maternal malnutrition and low birthweight.

We can find the p-value of the association by using the chi-square test as given by the following formula. This formula is appropriate only for a two-by-two table.

$$\text{Chi-square,} \; \chi^2 = \frac{n(ad - bc)^2}{(a+b)(c+d)(a+c)(b+d)}$$

The chi-square value that we have calculated from the data is 21.9 (note that in the formula above, n is the total number of cases and controls). The calculated chi-square value is then compared with the chi-square tabulated value.

For a two-by-two table, the tabulated chi-square value is 3.841 at the 95% confidence level with one degree of freedom (the degree of freedom for a chi-squared test in a two-by-two table is one). This value (3.841) is obtained from the chi-square distribution table, commonly found in standard statistics books or online. The p-value for the chi-square test is found to be less than 0.001. A p-value of less than 0.05 is considered statistically significant at the 95% confidence level.

Now, we have all the information (OR, 95% CI of OR, and p-value) that is needed to conclude the results. We can conclude from the data that malnourished women are 2.71 times more likely to deliver a low birthweight baby compared to well-nourished mothers, which is statistically significant at the 95% confidence level (OR: 2.71; 95% CI: 1.75 – 4.14; p<0.001).

If our calculated OR were 1.7 with a 95% CI of 0.87 – 2.51 (an interval that includes one), we would conclude that malnourished women are 1.7 times more likely to deliver a LBW baby compared to well-nourished women. However, this result is not statistically significant at the 95% confidence level (OR = 1.7; 95% CI: 0.87 – 2.51; p > 0.05).

Suppose that a case-control study was conducted to examine the effectiveness of a measles vaccine among children. The study shows that the OR for measles, if children are vaccinated compared to those who are not vaccinated, is 0.30 (95% CI: 0.21 – 0.42; p=0.02). When the OR is less than 1, we should conclude from the given data that vaccinated children are 70% [$(1-0.3) \times 100$] less likely to get measles compared to those who are not vaccinated, which is statistically significant (OR: 0.30; 95% CI: 0.21 – 0.42; p=0.02). In other words, the vaccine is 70% effective in preventing measles, or the vaccine provides 70% protection from getting measles infection.

7.8.3 Data Analysis of a Matched Case-Control Design

In a matched case-control design, cases are matched with controls for one or more factors (variables) one-by-one, and the status of exposure is noted. Data generated in such a design is presented in Table 7.3. It is important to note that the data presented in each cell of the table appears in pairs, as described below.

Cells "a" and "d" are called the *concordant pairs* as cases and controls are similar in terms of exposure, i.e., both cases and controls are either exposed (cell "a") or unexposed (cell "d"). These cells do not contribute to the data analysis. On the other hand, cells "b" and "c" are called the *discordant pairs*, as cases and controls are dissimilar in terms of the exposure of interest. For a matched-pair case-control design, OR is calculated by the following formula:

$$OR = \frac{\text{Cell in which cases are exposed}}{\text{Cells in which controls are exposed}} \quad \text{i.e.,} \quad \frac{b}{c} \qquad \left[\text{Formula 7.1}\right]$$

TABLE 7.3

Data presentation of a matched case-control design

		Control	
		Exposed	Unexposed
Case	Exposed	a	b
	Unexposed	c	d

- Data in cell "a" indicates both cases and controls are exposed;
- Data in cell "b" indicates cases are exposed while controls are unexposed;
- Data in cell "C" indicates cases are unexposed while controls are exposed; and
- Data in cell "d" indicates both cases and controls are unexposed.

However, if cases are placed on columns and controls on rows in a two-by-two table, the formula for the calculation of OR will be changed [OR will be equal to (c ÷ b)]. It is, therefore, suggested to remember the numerator (cell in which cases are exposed) and the denominator (cell in which controls are exposed) to avoid confusion.

The SE of lnOR for the matched-pair case-control study is calculated as:

$$\text{SE of lnOR} = \sqrt{\left(\frac{1}{b} + \frac{1}{c}\right)} \qquad\qquad \left[\text{Formula 7.2}\right]$$

With the SE of lnOR, we can calculate the 95% CI of OR by using the following formula:

$$95\% \text{ CI of OR} = \text{OR} \times e^{\pm(1.96 \times \text{SE of lnOR})} \qquad \left[\text{Formula 7.3}\right]$$

To determine the significance of the association (i.e., to get the p-value), we can use the chi-square test (called McNemar's test). The formula is as follows:

$$\text{Chi-square, } \chi^2 = \frac{\left(|b-c|-1\right)^2}{(b+c)} \qquad\qquad \left[\text{Formula 7.4}\right]$$

The two bars (before "b" and after "c") represent the absolute difference between "b" and "c", ignoring the negative sign.

Example

A matched case-control study was conducted to evaluate the effect of chewing betel quid (exposure) on oral cancer. Cases were histologically confirmed oral cancer cases, while controls were those who did not have oral cancer. Cases were matched with controls for gender. The study data are presented in Table 7.4.

TABLE 7.4

Data of a matched case-control study on oral cancer

		Control	
		Exposed	Unexposed
Case	Exposed	55 (a)	130 (b)
	Unexposed	75 (c)	100 (d)

To analyze the data, one cannot use the cells "a" and "d" since they are the concordant pairs. Using the formulas (Formulas 7.1 to 7.4), one can calculate the OR, SE of lnOR, 95% CI of OR, and the p-value, which are as follows:

$$OR = \frac{b}{c} = \frac{130}{75} = 1.73$$

The SE of lnOR = 0.15

The 95% CI of the OR is 1.30 – 2.30

$\chi^2 = 14.22$; p-value <0.01

The interpretation of the results is the same as discussed in Section 7.8.2. In this example, the calculated OR is greater than 1.0 (1.73), and the 95% CI does not include one. The p-value is also <0.05. We can, therefore, conclude that persons who chew betel quid are 1.73 times (or 73%) more likely to have oral cancer compared to those who do not chew betel quid, which is statistically significant at the 5% level of significance (OR: 1.73; 95% CI of OR: 1.30 – 2.30; p<0.01).

7.9 Relationship Between OR and RR

The relative risk (RR) is a direct measure of risk, while the OR is an indirect measure of risk. We can estimate the RR from the OR. The OR is a good estimate of the RR if the following assumptions are met.

- The incidence of the disease of interest is low (less than 10%). The OR tends to overestimate the RR if the incidence of a disease is high;
- Cases are representative of all cases in the community as regards to the exposure of interest; and

- Controls are representative of the general population (or non-diseased population) as regards to the exposure of interest.

If we calculate the OR from a cohort study, it (OR) will be equal to:

$$OR = \frac{\left(I^+\right) \div \left(1 - I^+\right)}{\left(I^-\right) \div \left(1 - I^-\right)} = RR \times \frac{\left(1 - I^-\right)}{\left(1 - I^+\right)}$$

Where I^+ represents the incidence of disease among exposed and I^- is the incidence of disease among unexposed.

The above equation indicates that the OR is a function of the RR and the quantity $[(1 - I^-) \div (1 - I^+)]$. The amount $[(1 - I^-) \div (1 - I^+)]$ is called the *biased fraction or in-built bias*. Therefore, the difference between the OR and the estimated RR depends on how big the biased fraction is. When disease incidence is low, this fraction is small, making the OR a close approximation of the RR (i.e., the OR becomes a good estimate of the RR). On the other hand, when disease incidence is high, the OR tends to overestimate the RR (away from the null value).

If it is felt that the OR exaggerates the RR, using the following formula, one can estimate the RR, provided the incidence among the unexposed (I^-) is known.

$$RR = \frac{OR}{1 - \left(I^-\right) + \left(I^- \times OR\right)} = \frac{OR}{1 - \left[\left(I^-\right) \times \left(1 - OR\right)\right]}$$

From the above formula, it is evident that the extent of variation between the RR and OR depends on the incidence of the disease among the unexposed group. An estimate of the incidence among the unexposed group can be obtained from other studies or from the same cohort study if it is a nested case-control design.

7.10 Potential Sources of Bias

Case-control studies are subjected to potential biases, which need to be kept in mind before interpreting the results and drawing conclusions from the study. The potential sources of bias in a case-control study include: a) selection bias; b) information (observation) bias; and c) misclassification bias (also see Chapter 15).

7.10.1 Selection Bias

Selection of an appropriate control group is always a challenge in case-control studies. Selection bias in case-control studies may occur due to the way cases and controls are selected for the study. For instance, in a hospital-based case-control study, if cases are selected from a hospital, they may not represent all cases in the community (Berksonian bias). Hospital cases may represent only those who survived and were referred for hospital care.

Similarly, if the hospital controls do not represent the general population in terms of exposure, this may introduce bias into the study. On the contrary, selecting controls from the community can also introduce selection bias if there is a high rate of nonresponse or unavailability of subjects (nonresponse bias), which may result in selecting controls from those who stay at home, such as the elderly, unemployed, or disabled people.

On the other hand, in a population-based case-control study, if the response rates for cases and controls are unequal (or low), it may introduce nonresponse bias into the study since it is usually found that those who agree to participate differ from those who do not participate.

7.10.2 Information Bias

In case-control studies, exposure information is commonly obtained by interviewing study subjects themselves or surrogates, such as a spouse, a close relative, or the parents of affected children. If the person interviewed knows the disease status, there is a greater probability of reporting an exposure compared to controls, which may introduce bias into the study. Similarly, if the study objectives and hypothesis are known to data collectors, knowledge about the disease status may influence the reporting and recording of the exposure of interest (interviewer bias).

The other form of information bias that can occur in case-control studies is recall bias. It is observed that cases are more likely to recall (remember) the events of past exposure than those who do not have the disease, leading to an overestimation of the effect.

7.10.3 Misclassification Bias

Misclassification indicates errors in categorizing the disease status or exposure status. Misclassification of cases (or controls) commonly occurs due to the inherent characteristics of the diagnostic test (sensitivity and specificity) used to classify cases and controls. Misclassification can occur as either *non-differential (or random) misclassification or differential misclassification.*

In non-differential misclassification, the same proportion of cases and controls are misclassified, while in differential misclassification, the proportions are different. Both forms of misclassification affect the estimates of an association, depending on the situation. The presence of non-differential misclassification underestimates the effect (risk) of an exposure on an outcome. In contrast, the presence of differential misclassification could either overestimate or underestimate the effects. However, in general, non-differential misclassification is believed to be less concerning than differential misclassification.

References

1.   Hennekens CH, Buring JE. *Epidemiology in Medicine*. 1st ed. Boston/ Toronto: Little Brown and Company; 1987.
2.   Gordis L. *Epidemiology*. 5th ed. Philadelphia: Elsevier Saunders; 2014.
3.   Schlesselman JJ, Stolley PD. *Case-Control Studies: Design, Conduct, Analysis*. New York: Oxford University Press; 1982.
4.   Lilienfeld DE, Stolley PD. *Foundations of Epidemiology*. 3rd ed. New York: Oxford University Press; 1994.
5.   Bonita R, Beaglehole R, Kjellström T. *Basic Epidemiology*. 2nd ed. Geneva: World Health Organization; 2006.
6.   Alexander LK, Lopes B, Ricchetti-Masterson K, Yeatts KB. *Case-Control Studies. ERIC Notebook*. 2nd ed. Chapel Hill, NC: UNC Gillings School of Global Public Health; 2015.
7.   Szklo M, Nieto FJ. *Epidemiology: Beyond the Basics*. 2nd ed. Boston: Jones and Bartlett Publishers; 2007.
8.   Fukai K, Furuya Y, Nakazawa S, Suzuki S, Takamoto I, Kobayashi N, et al. A case-control study of occupation and cardiovascular disease risk in Japanese men and women. *Sci Rep*. 2021;11:23983.
9.   Anderson LN, Heong SW, Chen Y, Thorpe KE, Adeli K, Howard A, et al. Vitamin D and fracture risk in early childhood: a case-control study. *Am J Epidemiol*. 2017;185(12):1255–62. doi: 10.1093/aje/kww204
10. Nguyen J, Le QH, Duong BH, Sun P, Pham HT. A matched case-control study of risk factors for breast cancer risk in Vietnam. *Int J Breast Cancer*. 2016;2016:7164623. https://doi.org/10.1155/2016/7164623
11. Pramanick S, Chakraborty D, Bera S , Roy A, Mukhopadhyay S. A case-control study on risk factors of breast cancer among women attending a tertiary care hospital in Kolkata, India. *J Cell Biol Cell Metab*. 2020;7:020. doi:10.24966/CBCM-1943/100020

8

Cohort Studies

Mohammad Tajul Islam

Cohort studies are important observational analytical study designs in epidemiology to ascertain the cause (or a risk factor) for an outcome (e.g., a disease). Cohort studies are also called prospective, longitudinal, or forward-looking studies. This design provides an opportunity to directly measure the incidence of disease among exposed and unexposed groups as well as the relative risk (RR). Relative risk is a direct measure of risk and indicates the strength of the association between exposure and outcome [1–7].

8.1 Design

Cohort studies always begin with exposure. The basic difference in the designs of cohort and case-control studies is that cohort studies begin with exposure, while case-control studies begin with outcome.

In cohort studies, at the beginning, a group or groups of individuals are defined on the basis of exposure (such as exposed and unexposed) to a suspected risk factor for a disease. In cohort studies, all study subjects (both exposed and unexposed) must be free from the disease of interest at the beginning. After the exposure status is defined, all individuals are followed over a certain period of time to observe the occurrence of the outcome (disease) of interest [1–5].

Because of the design, cohort studies have a number of advantages. The major advantages of cohort studies are that the temporal relationship between exposure and outcome can be clearly established since subjects are free from the disease of interest at the time of defining the exposure status, and cohort studies tend to minimize the potential for selection bias. However, there are several limitations of cohort studies. Since cohort studies require follow-up of a large number of people, they are expensive and time-consuming, and they have the potential bias associated with losses to follow-up, especially when the follow-up period is long. All these potential problems must be carefully considered when designing and conducting a cohort study. Details about the advantages and limitations of cohort studies are discussed in Chapter 4.

8.1.1 Types of Cohort Studies

Cohort studies can be classified based on the timing of identification and follow-up of exposed and unexposed groups as follows:

a)   Prospective or concurrent cohort studies;

b)   Retrospective, non-concurrent, or historical cohort studies; and

c)   Ambidirectional cohort studies.

In prospective or concurrent cohort studies, the exposure status is defined as exposed and unexposed at the *present time* in a group or groups of individuals who are free from the disease of interest at the beginning (Chapter 4; Figure 4.4). The groups are then followed (from the present time) over a period of time in the future to ascertain the occurrence of the outcome of interest in both groups. Therefore, at the time of initiation of a prospective cohort study, the outcome has not yet occurred.

Retrospective or non-concurrent cohort studies begin *before the present time* by defining the exposure status (exposed and unexposed) of a group or groups of individuals, commonly using the past records (Chapter 4; Figure 4.5). The occurrence of the outcome in both groups is ascertained at the present time through interviews, medical record reviews, or other means. Therefore, in retrospective cohort studies, both exposure and the outcome of interest have already occurred when the study is initiated.

The basic difference between prospective and retrospective cohort studies is the time of initiating the study. Prospective cohort studies begin at the present time with the exposure, while retrospective cohort studies begin before the present time and, of course, with the exposure (Chapter 4; Figures 4.4 and 4.5).

The major advantage of retrospective cohort studies is that they can be conducted much more quickly and cheaply compared to prospective cohort studies (since both exposure and outcome have already occurred). However, retrospective cohort studies depend on the availability of exposure data in sufficient detail from previous records. Since data are not commonly recorded for the purpose of testing a specific hypothesis, in most cases, data remain incomplete and non-comparable for the study subjects. Moreover, information on potential confounding factors, such as dietary and smoking habits, physical exercise, and other lifestyle characteristics, may not be available from the records for adjustment. In contrast, in prospective cohort studies, the investigator has the opportunity to obtain complete information on both exposure and confounding factors from study subjects at the beginning of the study [1, 2].

In ambidirectional cohort designs, data are collected both retrospectively and prospectively on the same cohort. Such a design can be used to determine the short-term and long-term effects of an exposure on an outcome.

Sometimes, case-control studies are designed within an ongoing cohort study, called nested case-control designs [8]. Using nested case-control designs, one can evaluate the risk factors for an outcome at a lower cost. Such a study design also confirms the precedence of exposure for an outcome. This study design is further discussed in Section 7.2.2.

8.2 Selection of Study Subjects

The basic principle of selecting the study population for a cohort study is to identify a group of people who are exposed to one or more suspected risk factors and another group who are not exposed. All individuals must be free from the outcome of interest at baseline (i.e., at the beginning of the study). The exposed and unexposed groups can be selected from different population sources depending on feasibility and scientific considerations, including the ease of obtaining information from the study subjects [1–3].

8.2.1 Selection of Exposed Group

When the prevalence of exposure is high in the general population, such as smoking habits, alcohol consumption, or chewing betel quid, a sufficient number of exposed (as well as unexposed) individuals can be obtained from a geographically and demographically defined population. Information on exposures can be obtained at baseline by taking a sample (or the whole population) from such a population and examining them periodically in the future to ascertain the occurrence of outcomes. This is the best choice for the investigation of a number of common risk factors (e.g., smoking, hypertension, or alcohol consumption) for relatively common outcomes (e.g., coronary heart disease, stroke, or cirrhosis of the liver). Such a strategy of selecting the study subjects from a population (general cohort) was adopted in the well-known Framingham Heart Study in the US [2, 9, 10]. The use of a general cohort allows the researchers to study the effects of a variety of risk factors on different outcomes. For example, the Framingham Heart Study, which is a population-based observational cohort study, began in 1948 by recruiting 5,127 (about two-thirds of the population of the town) men and women aged between 30 and 62 years from the town of Framingham, Massachusetts, USA [2]. Information on suspected risk factors was collected from all the study subjects at baseline (after excluding the outcomes of interest) and classified into exposed and unexposed groups. The study subjects were then followed and assessed every two years to ascertain the occurrence of outcomes of interest.

For rare exposures, such as exposure to asbestos or X-ray radiation, it is very difficult to obtain a sufficient number of exposed individuals from the general population. In such a situation, it is convenient to select the exposed group from individuals who are exposed due to their occupations, such as workers in asbestos factories or the radiology department of hospitals.

8.2.2 Selection of Unexposed Group

A comparison (unexposed) group is needed to test hypotheses. The selection of a comparison group is always a challenge. Ideally, the unexposed group should be as similar as possible to the exposed group with regard to all other factors that may influence the occurrence of the outcome except for the exposure of interest. There are several options for selecting the unexposed group for a cohort study.

In cohort studies, where a single group is selected from a population (general cohort, as cited above), the unexposed individuals can be utilized as the comparison group, as considered in Framingham's study [2, 9, 10]. In this study, a sample of 5,127 individuals was selected randomly from the general population. The subjects were then classified into exposed and unexposed groups based on their specific exposure status (e.g., smoking habit, hypertension, or serum cholesterol level).

In cohort studies of special exposure groups (rare exposure), such as occupational exposure to asbestos, the comparison group may be selected from the community where the exposed individuals live or from the workers of another factory (e.g., a cotton industry). The comparison group for such an occupational exposure can also be selected from the workers of the same industry who do a different type of job (e.g., an administrative job) and are not exposed to the risk factor of interest.

Sometimes, the incidence of a disease in an occupationally exposed group is compared with the incidence of the disease in the general population after adjusting for age and sex. Such a comparison is acceptable when the prevalence of the exposure of interest in the general population is very low (e.g., exposure to asbestos). However, such a comparison may be subject to bias, called the *healthy worker effect* (see Chapter 15).

In summary, the study subjects (exposed and unexposed individuals) for a cohort study can be selected in either of the following ways:

> First, select a defined population or take a sample from the population (where some are already exposed to the suspected risk factor) before their exposure status is identified. This strategy is suitable when the

prevalence of exposure is high in the general population (e.g., prevalence of smoking). Once the study subjects are selected from the defined population, individuals are classified as exposed and unexposed by taking a history, performing blood tests, or using other methods. The Framingham Heart Study, as cited earlier, used this strategy to select the study subjects.

Second, selecting a group of individuals on the basis of whether or not they are already exposed. Such a strategy is suitable for rare exposures, such as occupationally exposed cohorts. For example, to test the hypothesis that exposure to asbestos is a risk factor for lung cancer, a researcher may select a group of people from an asbestos industry as an exposed group and another group of people who are not exposed from a cotton industry.

Third, occasionally, a defined population is selected before they are exposed to the suspected risk factor, but the exposure status is determined during the initial follow-up period. For example, to study the relationship between alcohol consumption and oral cancer, a population of primary school children may be identified and followed. About ten to 15 years later, when they are in their teens, the students are identified as those who consume alcohol (exposed) and those who do not (unexposed). These groups are then followed for another ten to 20 years (the latent period for oral cancer) to observe the incidence rates of oral cancer in both groups for comparison. This method of selecting study subjects requires an even longer time to complete the study.

8.3 Information on Exposure and Outcome

Information on exposure, outcome, and potential confounding factors is needed for data analyses to find associations between exposure and outcome. The ability to accurately collect relevant information from the exposed and unexposed groups is crucial for the validity of the study.

Information on exposure can be obtained from a number of sources, such as: a) directly from the study subjects through questionnaire interviews, physical examinations, or laboratory tests; b) from the available medical or employment records; or c) direct measurement of the environment in which the study subjects have lived or worked.

Similarly, the outcome information can be obtained directly from the study subjects (through questionnaire interviews, physical examinations, or laboratory tests) and from available medical records (e.g., periodic health examinations or hospital records), including death certificates. Outcome information can also be obtained with the use of standardized diagnostic procedures applied to all subjects. Commonly, a combination of various sources of data is used to obtain complete information.

However, each of the sources of information has its own advantages and limitations that need to be considered while selecting the source of information on exposure and outcome for the study. Utilization of data from different sources depends on the study objective and hypothesis. It is always advantageous to utilize the available sources of information (if reliable) as much as possible and collect additional information from individuals as needed. Further details about information collection on exposure and outcome can be found elsewhere [1–3].

8.4 Follow-Up of Study Subjects

All individuals enrolled in the cohort study need to be followed from the beginning of the study (in concurrent cohort studies) to the future to observe the occurrence of the outcome of interest. How long the study subjects will be followed depends on the length of the latency period for the outcome. The length of follow-up may be short (e.g., studies to observe the outcome of pneumonia in children) or long (e.g., studies related to chronic disease outcomes like cancer, hypertension, or heart disease). The follow-up of individuals in a cohort study is always a challenge, especially if the follow-up period is long. In cohort studies, a complete follow-up of all individuals, whether exposed or unexposed, should be the goal.

In cohort studies, particularly when the follow-up period is long, loss of study subjects to follow-up is very common. Losses to follow-up may occur because of outmigration, death due to other causes than those of interest, or withdrawal from the study. In general, the longer the follow-up period, the more difficult it is to get complete follow-up data from all subjects. Failure to obtain outcome information from a substantial proportion (more than 30%) of subjects (exposed or unexposed) is a major source of bias in cohort studies and makes the interpretation of results difficult [1].

8.5 Data Analysis

Data from cohort studies are analyzed in terms of incidence of disease among exposed and unexposed groups and relative risk or risk ratio (RR), including the confidence interval, in order to determine the association between exposure and disease. The disease incidence and RR can also be calculated for various levels of exposure (e.g., for mild, moderate, and heavy smoking) to assess the dose-response relationship as well as a combination of factors. The other measures of association that can be calculated from the data of cohort studies include attributable risk (AR), proportional attributable risk (%AR), and population attributable risk (PAR).

Example
A cohort study is designed to test the hypothesis of whether or not drinking alcohol is a risk factor for stomach cancer. To test the hypothesis, 2,000 individuals who drink alcohol (exposed) and another 2,000 individuals who do not drink alcohol (unexposed) were identified from a population. All the study subjects were free of stomach cancer at the beginning and were followed for a period of ten years. Data obtained from the study is given in Table 8.1.

From the data, we can calculate the cumulative incidence of stomach cancer in exposed (who consume alcohol) and unexposed (who do not consume alcohol) groups. Cumulative incidence is the measure of an individual's risk of developing the disease. We can also calculate the relative risk (RR), which is a direct measure of risk, to determine the strength of the association between alcohol consumption and stomach cancer. The cumulative incidence is calculated as:

$$\text{Cumulative incidence} = \frac{\text{No. of people developed the disease}}{\text{No. of people at risk at the beginning}}$$

Therefore (using symbols of Table 8.1),

$$\text{Cumulative incidence in exposed} = \frac{a}{(a+b)} \text{ or } \frac{58}{2,000} = 0.029 \text{ or } 2.90\%$$

and

$$\text{Cumulative incidence in unexposed} = \frac{c}{(c+d)} \text{ or } \frac{35}{2,000} = 0.0175 \text{ or } 1.75\%$$

TABLE 8.1

Frequency distribution of stomach cancer by alcohol consumption

	Stomach Cancer		
	Present	Absent	Total
Drink alcohol	58 (a)	1,942 (b)	2,000 (a + b)
Don't drink alcohol	35 (c)	1,965 (d)	2,000 (c + d)
Total	93 (a + c)	3,907 (b + d)	4,000 (n)

Data indicate that the cumulative incidence of stomach cancer in the exposed group (2.90% over a period of ten years) is higher than the cumulative incidence in the unexposed group (1.75% over a period of ten years). This information suggests that exposure may be associated with the development of stomach cancer since incidence is higher in the exposed group. Now, to calculate the RR, use the following formula:

$$\text{Relative risk}\,(\text{RR}) = \frac{\text{Cumulative Incidence in exposed}}{\text{Cumulative Incidence in unexposed}} \text{ or } \frac{2.90}{1.75} = 1.66$$

8.5.1 Interpretation of Relative Risk

Relative risk indicates the amount of risk associated with exposure for the development of an outcome. When the incidence among the exposed is greater than the incidence among the unexposed, the RR will be greater than one. Therefore, an RR greater than one suggests that exposure is associated with a higher risk of developing the disease (i.e., exposure is a risk factor for the disease). In contrast, an RR of less than one indicates that exposure is associated with a lower incidence (risk) of disease than being unexposed. This means that exposure provides some kind of protection from developing the disease (i.e., exposure is a protective factor). When RR is equal to one (also called the null value), the incidences among exposed and unexposed groups are the same, indicating there is no association between exposure and disease.

In our example, RR is 1.66, indicating that individuals who consume alcohol are at 1.66 times higher risk of developing stomach cancer compared to those who do not consume alcohol. As we are not sure whether the calculated RR (1.66) is by chance or not (i.e., because of the random error or not), we need to calculate the confidence interval (CI) of the RR. In health research, we prefer the 95% CI. The 95% CI of RR can be calculated by using the following formula.

$$95\% \text{ CI of RR} = \text{RR} \times e^{\pm(1.96 \times \text{SE of lnRR})}$$

Where "SE" represents the standard error and "lnRR" indicates the natural log of RR (also see Section 7.8.2).

The SE of lnRR can be calculated by using the following formula:

$$\text{SE}\,(\text{standard error}) \text{ of lnRR} = \sqrt{\left(\frac{1}{a} - \frac{1}{a+b} + \frac{1}{c} - \frac{1}{c+d}\right)}$$

In our example, the SE of lnRR is 0.21, as shown below:

$$\text{SE of lnRR} = \sqrt{\left(\frac{1}{82} - \frac{1}{2000} + \frac{1}{35} - \frac{1}{2000}\right)} = 0.21$$

Therefore, the 95% CI of RR is 1.10 – 2.51 as shown below (using a scientific calculator, one can find these values):

$$95\% \text{ CI of RR} = 1.66 \times e^{\pm(1.96 \times 0.21)} = 1.10 - 2.51$$

If the 95% CI of the RR includes one (i.e., if one falls within the range of the 95% CI), the RR is not statistically significant (i.e., the result may be by chance), indicating no association between exposure and outcome. In our example, the 95% CI for RR is 1.10 – 2.51, and the range does not include one. Therefore, there is a significant association between alcohol consumption and stomach cancer. Moreover, as the whole range is greater than one, exposure is a risk factor for the outcome. If both lower and upper values of the 95% CI were less than one, it would be a protective factor. We can find the *p-value* of the association by applying the chi-square test as given by the following formula (this formula is appropriate only for a two-by-two table):

$$\text{Chi-square, } \chi^2 = \frac{n(ad - bc)^2}{(a+b)(c+d)(a+c)(b+d)}$$

i.e.,

$$\text{Chi-square, } \chi^2 = \frac{4000 \times [(58 \times 1965) - (35 \times 1942)]^2}{(2000 \times 2000 \times 93 \times 3907)} = 5.82$$

The chi-square calculated value of our data is 5.82, which is greater than the chi-square tabulated value of 3.841 at the 95% confidence level and one degree of freedom (obtained from the chi-square distribution table). The *p-value* for the chi-square test is 0.015, which is statistically significant (since it is less than 0.05).

Now, to conclude the results, it can be said that individuals who consume alcohol are at 1.66 times higher risk of developing stomach cancer compared to those who do not consume alcohol, which is statistically significant at the 95% confidence level (RR: 1.66; 95% CI: 1.10 – 2.51; p= 0.015).

How do we interpret an RR when it is less than one, for example, 0.80? If the RR is 0.80 (95% CI: 0.70 – 0.95), this suggests that exposure is associated with a 20% reduction in the incidence (or a 20% risk reduction) of the outcome (1 – 0.80 = 0.20 or 20%). In other words, exposure provides 20% protection against developing the disease. Since the 95% CI does not include one, the RR is also statistically significant. Thus, exposed individuals have a 20% lower risk of developing the disease compared to those who are not exposed.

It is important to note that RR indicates the strength of the association, while the *p-value* indicates the Type I error that has been committed in the study. A smaller *p-value* indicates stronger evidence of an association between exposure and outcome, but not the strength of the association.

8.6 Calculation of Risk When the Measurement of Observation Is Person-Time

When the measurement of observation is person-time, we calculate the incidence rate (also called incidence density or ID) and the incidence rate ratio (IRR), including its 95% CI. Person-time observation is used when study subjects are lost to follow-up or when individuals are observed for varying lengths of time in a study (see Section 3.3). For example, two groups of people, smokers (exposed) and non-smokers (unexposed), were followed for a period of ten years, and the observation was measured in terms of person-years. The outcome of interest was oral cancer. Information obtained from the cohort study is given in Table 8.2.

From the data, we can calculate the incidence rates (IR) of oral cancer among smokers and non-smokers, as well as the incidence rate ratio (IRR) as follows:

$$\text{IR in exposed (smokers)} = \frac{75}{20,000} \times 1,000 = 3.75 \text{ per } 1,000 \text{ person} - \text{years}$$

$$\text{IR in unexposed (non} - \text{smokers)} = \frac{35}{25,000} \times 1,000 = 1.4 \text{ per } 1,000 \text{ person} - \text{years}$$

Therefore, the incidence rate ratio (IRR) is

TABLE 8.2

Distribution of oral cancer cases and person-time of observations

	Oral cancer	Person-year
Smoker	75 (a)	20,000 (n1)
Non-smoker	35 (c)	25,000 (n2)
Total	110 (D)	45,000 (N)

$$\text{IRR} = \frac{\text{IR in exposed (smokers)}}{\text{IR in unexposed (non-smokers)}} \quad \text{i.e.,} \quad \frac{3.75}{1.40} = 2.68$$

The interpretation of IRR is similar to that of RR, as previously discussed. When the IRR is greater than one, exposure is a risk factor. If the IRR is less than one, exposure is a protective factor, and if the IRR is equal to one, there is no association between exposure and outcome. In our example, exposure (smoking) seems to be a risk factor for oral cancer since the IRR is greater than one. However, we need to calculate the 95% CI of the IRR to prove that it is not by chance. The 95% CI of the IRR can be calculated by using the following formula (SE: standard error; lnIRR: natural log of IRR):

$$95\% \text{ CI of IRR} = \text{IRR} \times e^{\pm(1.96 \times \text{SE of lnIRR})}$$

The SE of lnIRR is given by the following formula (assuming a Poisson distribution):

$$\text{SE of lnIRR} = \sqrt{\left(\frac{1}{a} + \frac{1}{c}\right)}$$

In our example, the SE of lnIRR is 0.20 as shown below.

$$\text{SE of lnIRR} = \sqrt{\left(\frac{1}{75} + \frac{1}{35}\right)} = 0.20$$

Therefore, the 95% CI of IRR is:

$$95\% \text{ CI of IRR} = 2.68 \times e^{\pm(1.96 \times 0.20)} = 1.81 - 3.97$$

Finally, to find the p-value, we will use the chi-square test, the formula (using the symbols of Table 8.2) of which is:

$$\text{Chi-square, } \chi^2 = \frac{\left[a - (n1 \times D \div N)\right]^2}{(D \times n1 \times n2 \div N^2)}$$

In our example, the calculated chi-square value is 25.1, which is greater than the chi-square tabulated value of 3.841 at a 95% confidence level and one degree of freedom (obtained from the chi-square distribution table). The p-value of the test is <0.001. Since the p-value is less than 0.05, there is a significant association between smoking and oral cancer.

Given all the information, we can conclude that smokers have a 2.68 times higher rate of developing oral cancer compared to non-smokers, which is statistically significant at the 95% confidence level (IRR: 2.68; 95% CI: 1.81 – 3.97; p<0.001).

8.7 Attributable Risk

Another measure of risk in epidemiology is the attributable risk, or risk difference, which indicates the amount of disease incidence attributable to a specific risk factor. Other measures that are calculated from the data of a cohort study include the proportional or percent attributable risk (%AR) and the population attributable risk (PAR). The PAR is particularly important in public health as it provides information about the expected reduction in disease incidence in the population if the risk factor is eliminated. We will calculate these measures using the cumulative incidences in the exposed (2.90%) and unexposed (1.75%) groups, as well as the RR (1.66), which were calculated based on data in Table 8.1.

8.7.1 Attributable Risk or Risk Difference

The attributable risk (AR), or risk difference, is the difference in the incidence of disease between exposed and unexposed groups. It is calculated by subtracting the incidence of disease in the unexposed group from the incidence of disease in the exposed group. The incidence of disease in unexposed individuals is sometimes referred to as the *baseline risk*. The AR indicates the amount of greater risk (incidence) attributable to exposure in the exposed group.

$$\text{Attributable risk}\left(\text{AR}\right) = \text{Incidence in exposed} - \text{Incidence in unexposed}$$

In our example, the AR is 1.15% (2.90% – 1.75%). This indicates that individuals who drink alcohol experience a 1.15% higher incidence of stomach cancer than those who do not drink alcohol.

8.7.2 Proportional or Percent Attributable Risk

The proportional attributable risk (%AR) indicates what proportion (%) of the total incidence of disease in the exposed group is attributable to the risk factor and is calculated as:

$$\%AR = \frac{\text{Incidence in exposed} - \text{Incidence in unexposed}}{\text{Incidence in exposed}} \text{ or, } \frac{RR-1}{RR}$$

In our example, the %AR is 0.397 [(2.90 – 1.75) ÷ 2.90], or 39.7%. It indicates that alcohol consumption (the exposure) is responsible for 39.7% of stomach cancer cases among individuals who consume alcohol (exposed). In other words, 39.7% of stomach cancer cases among those who consume alcohol could have been prevented if they had stopped drinking alcohol.

8.7.3 Population Attributable Risk

Population attributable risk (PAR), also called attributable fraction or etiologic fraction, is an important measure of risk in epidemiology. The PAR answers the question: if exposure (e.g., drinking alcohol) were eliminated from the population, what proportion of disease incidence (e.g., stomach cancer) in the total population could be prevented? To calculate the PAR, first, we need to calculate the incidence of disease in the total population, which requires information on the proportion of the population exposed to the risk factor of interest (i.e., the prevalence of the risk factor in the population).

We will calculate the incidence of stomach cancer in the total population and the PAR using the cumulative incidences in the exposed (2.90%) and unexposed (1.75%) groups, along with the RR (1.66), as calculated earlier from the data in Table 8.1. Let us assume that 20% (0.20) of the general population from which the study subjects were selected consumes alcohol. The incidence of disease in the total population is calculated as:

$$\text{Incidence in pop.} = \left[P \times \text{Incidence in exposed} \right] + \left[Q \times \text{Incidence in unexposed} \right]$$

Where P is the proportion of the population exposed to the risk factor (i.e., consumes alcohol) and Q is (1 – P).

Therefore, the incidence of stomach cancer in the total population is:

$$\text{Incidence in population} = \left[0.20 \times 2.90 \right] + \left[0.80 \times 1.75 \right] = 1.98\%$$

Once we have the data on the incidence of disease in the population, the PAR can be calculated using the following formula:

$$PAR = \frac{\text{Incidence in the population} - \text{Incidence in unexposed}}{\text{Incidence in the population}}$$

$$PAR = \frac{1.98 - 1.75}{1.98} \times 100 = 11.6\%$$

The alternative formula for the calculation of PAR is:

$$PAR = \frac{P \times (RR - 1)}{[P \times (RR - 1)] + 1}$$

Where P represents the proportion of the population exposed to the risk factor.

Population-attributable risk (PAR) indicates the potential impact of public health interventions on the outcome of interest. In our example, the PAR is 11.6%, meaning that if it were possible to eliminate alcohol consumption (exposure) in the population, the incidence of stomach cancer in the entire population would decrease by 11.6%.

8.8 Potential Sources of Bias in Cohort Studies

Cohort studies are subject to a number of potential biases. These biases must be either avoided or taken into consideration while conducting cohort studies. The presence of bias can make the interpretation of study results difficult. The major types of bias that may affect cohort studies are discussed below (also see Chapter 15).

8.8.1 Bias in the Assessment of Outcome

Persons who assess the outcome, if they know the exposure status of individuals as well as the hypothesis being tested, may introduce bias during the ascertainment of disease. Persons who assess the outcome may have a greater tendency to identify disease among those who are exposed than the unexposed. This type of bias can be minimized by blinding data collectors to the study hypothesis and the exposure status of participants. Another way to introduce bias in the assessment of an outcome is the use of different instruments or criteria to ascertain the outcome for the exposed and unexposed individuals.

8.8.2 Information Bias

If the quality and extent of information obtained differ between exposed and unexposed groups, this may introduce significant bias in the study. Such problems are more likely to occur in historical cohort studies, where information is obtained from past records that are mostly incomplete and inconsistent.

8.8.3 Nonresponse and Nonparticipation Bias

Nonresponse and nonparticipation can introduce significant bias and complicate the interpretation of the study findings. Similarly, failure to follow-up can be a serious problem. If people with the disease are selectively lost to follow-up, the incidence rates calculated in the exposed and unexposed groups will be clearly difficult to interpret. Therefore, cohort studies should aim to achieve complete follow-up of all study participants, both exposed and unexposed, throughout the study period.

References

1. Hennekens CH, Buring JE. *Epidemiology in Medicine*. Boston/Toronto: Little, Brown and Company; 1987.
2. Gordis L. *Epidemiology*. 5th ed. Philadelphia: Elsevier Saunders; 2014.
3. Lilienfeld DE, Stolley PD. *Foundations of Epidemiology*. 3rd ed. New York: Oxford University Press; 1994.
4. Ibrahim M, Alexander L, Shy C, Farr S. Cohort studies. *UNC School of Public Health: ERIC Notebook*. 1999;3:1–3.
5. Bonita R, Beaglehole R, Kjellström T. *Basic Epidemiology*. 2nd ed. Geneva: World Health Organization; 2006.
6. Setia MS. Methodology series module 1: Cohort studies. *Indian J Dermatol*. 2016;61(1):21–5. doi:10.4103/0019-5154.174011.
7. Wang X, Kattan MW. Cohort studies: Design, analysis, and reporting. *CHEST*. 2020;158(1S):S72–S78. doi:10. 1016/j.chest.2020.03.016.
8. Szklo M, Nieto FJ. *Epidemiology: Beyond the Basics*. 2nd ed. Boston: Jones and Bartlett Publishers; 2007.
9. Framingham Heart Study. [Internet] [cited 2022 Dec 13]. Available from: www.framinghamheartstudy.org/
10. Stroke and Cerebrovascular Center. *Framingham Study* [Internet] [cited 2022 Dec 13]. Available from: www.bmc.org/stroke-and-cerebrovascular-center/research/framingham-study

9

Clinical Trials

Mohammad Tajul Islam

Experimental studies are concerned with the evaluation of the efficacy of interventions. Experimental studies are conducted either in a clinical setting or in the community. Experimental designs are mainly of three types: clinical trials, community trials, and field trials (Section 4.1.2.2). Field trials are designed to assess the effectiveness of preventive interventions for diseases, such as vaccination (e.g., for the prevention of measles) or health education aimed at preventing diseases (e.g., diarrhea) through behavior change.

Over the past decades, randomized clinical and community trials have been recognized as the preferred method for evaluating medical and community interventions. In this chapter, the basic principles of clinical trial designs are discussed. More details about clinical trials are described elsewhere [1, 2].

9.1 Clinical Trials

A clinical trial is defined as "a prospective study comparing the effects and value of intervention(s) against a control group in human beings" [1]. Clinical trials are experimental studies that are analogous to cohort studies. In clinical trials, subjects must be followed forward for a certain period of time from the point of enrollment. Clinical trials are always prospective and cannot be retrospective. It is not necessary that all subjects be followed for the same period of time or enrolled in the study at the same point in a clinical trial.

The main objective of clinical trials is to generate ideas for improving treatment. Clinical trials should include a control group (controlled trials). The control group, receiving the standard treatment or a placebo, should be similar to the patients in the treatment group. If there is no standard treatment available of any real value, the control group may remain either untreated or given a placebo.

DOI: 10.1201/9781003654803-9"

To obtain an unbiased evaluation of the efficacy of a treatment, each patient needs to be randomly assigned (a randomized trial) either to the new treatment or the standard treatment (or placebo). Blinding clinical trials are another approach for achieving an unbiased evaluation. A properly planned and conducted clinical trial provides the best evidence for the evaluation of the efficacy and safety of a new treatment or intervention.

The basic steps for a clinical trial are a) clearly state the objectives and hypotheses; b) develop a detailed written protocol; c) conduct the trial carefully in accordance with the protocol; d) analyze the data to test the hypotheses using appropriate statistical methods; and e) draw conclusions and publish results (Figure 9.1). A protocol must always be written before organizing a clinical trial. The protocol is a guide for the researchers, which should be followed while conducting the study.

9.2 Clinical Trial Phases

Clinical trials of a new drug conducted under the sponsorship of pharmaceutical companies follow four phases to establish the efficacy of the drug [1–4]. These phases are generally guidelines and may not be taken as mandatory rules [1].

Phase I: Clinical pharmacology and toxicity

The objective of Phase I trials is to study the safety (not efficacy) of a drug. In this phase, trials are performed on human volunteers to determine the acceptable single dose of the drug (i.e., how much drug can be given without causing any serious side effects). Drug metabolism is also studied in this phase. After the trial on volunteers, the Phase I trial is extended to patients on a small scale, usually involving around 20–80 patients.

Phase II: Initial treatment effect

In this phase, further evaluation of the safety and efficacy of the new drug is conducted in 100–300 patients. If the drug passes the Phase II trial, it is then tested in Phase III.

Phase III: Full-scale evaluation of treatment

After a drug is found to be effective in a Phase II trial, a full-scale trial is given to assess the efficacy of the new drug in a substantial number of patients (1,000 to 3,000 or more). The clinical trials that we see in scientific clinical investigations fall into this phase.

Phase IV: Post-marketing surveillance

This phase begins after the drug is approved for use. This is the long-term phase, where follow-up is undertaken to monitor the adverse effects and long-term morbidities and mortalities.

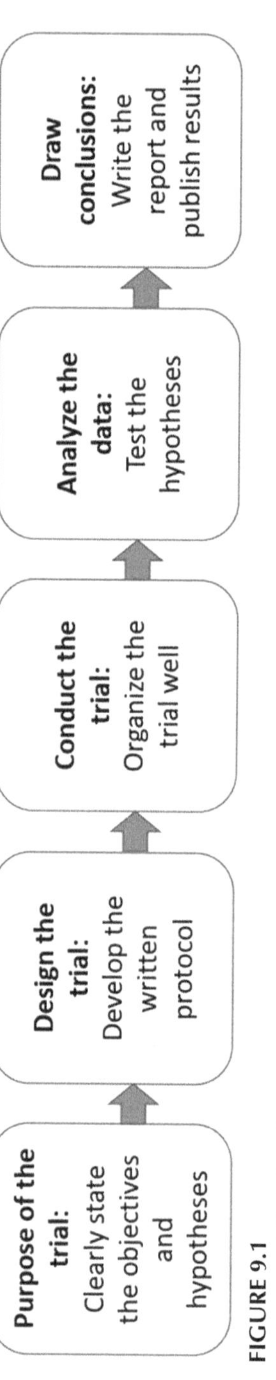

FIGURE 9.1
Basic steps of clinical trials.

9.3 Study Protocol

A study protocol is always needed for a well-designed clinical trial. A research protocol is a written document that presents a detailed plan for how to conduct the study. It is the written guide for researchers, caregivers, and evaluators involved in the study. It is also viewed as a written agreement between investigators and patients. The protocol should provide detailed information about the background, objectives, hypotheses, study design, methodology, statistical considerations, and organization of the trial. The study protocol should include sufficient detail so that anyone reading it can understand the methods and replicate the study. It should be developed during the planning phase before the enrollment of patients in the study.

Many protocols are now available in published journals. The main features of a protocol, as suggested by Pocock [2], are provided in Box 9.1. Note that this is a rough guide and may need to be adapted depending on the circumstances of the trial. Further details about writing a protocol can be seen in the book edited by Pocock [2].

9.4 Trial Designs

The basic design of clinical trials is shown in Figure 9.2. Clinical trials begin with the selection of eligible subjects. After obtaining informed consent, eligible subjects are randomized to receive either the new treatment or the standard treatment (or placebo). The study subjects in each group are followed over time to observe how many have improved in the new treatment group and in the standard treatment group. Data are then statistically analyzed to compare the outcome differences in order to conclude the results. The frequently used design options for a clinical trial is discussed below.

BOX 9.1   MAIN FEATURES OF A CLINICAL TRIAL PROTOCOL

• Background and rationale	• Registration and randomization of patients
• Study objective: General and specific objectives	• Treatment schedule
• Hypothesis	• Protocol deviation
• Trial design	• Methods of patient evaluation
• Sample size	• Monitoring of trial progress
• Patient enrolment criteria including the exclusion criteria	• Forms and data management
• Patient consent	• Plans for data analysis
	• Administrative responsibilities

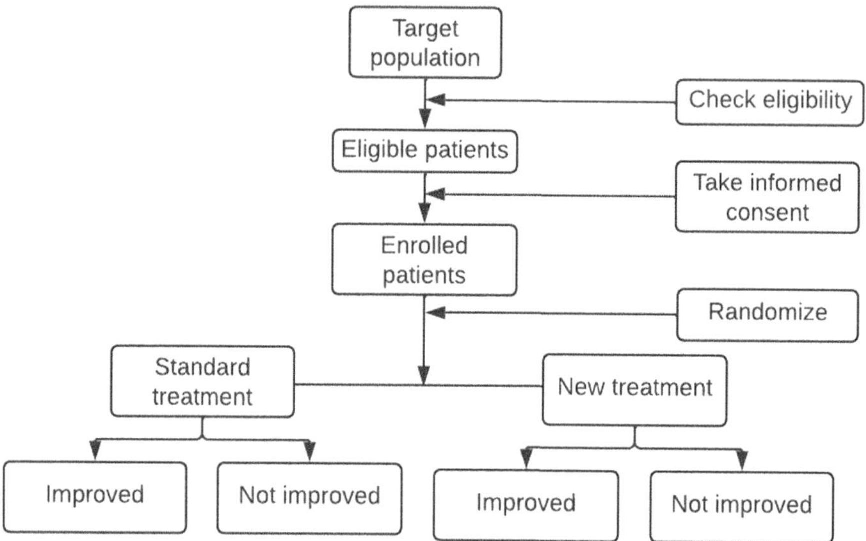

FIGURE 9.2
Randomized trial design.

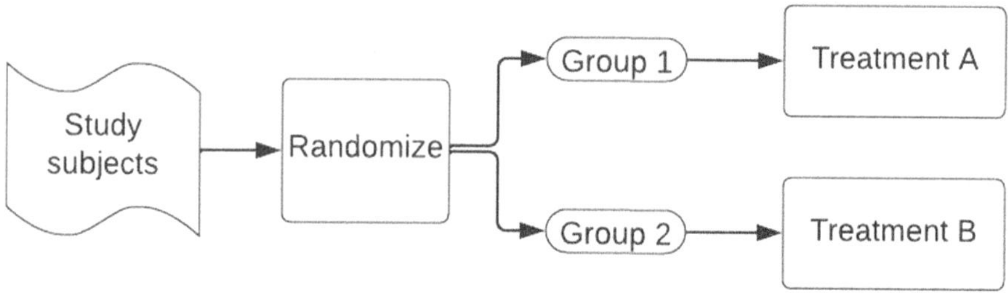

FIGURE 9.3
Parallel group design.

9.4.1 Parallel Group Design

The simplest and most commonly used design in clinical trials is the parallel group design. In this design, two (or more) different groups of patients are studied simultaneously – one group receives the new treatment, while the other group receives the standard treatment or a placebo (Figure 9.3). Once study participants have been randomized and assigned to a study group, they cannot be reassigned to another group for the duration of the study. These groups are followed for a certain period of time, and improvements in outcome in the new treatment group are compared with the improvements in outcome in the standard treatment group to conclude the results.

9.4.2 Crossover Design

Crossover designs are useful and can be employed in clinical trials to study short-term responses. In crossover designs, every patient participating in the clinical trial receives both treatment A (e.g., the new treatment; Group 1) and treatment B (e.g., the standard treatment or placebo; Group 2) for equal periods of time but in a different order. For instance, Group 1 might receive treatment A first, followed by treatment B, while Group 2 receives treatment B first, followed by treatment A. The order of treatments can be decided randomly. The major advantages of crossover designs are: a) each patient acts as their own control, thus balancing for factors that may influence the outcome, and b) crossover designs require a smaller sample size.

Crossovers in a trial may be *planned or unplanned*. In planned crossover designs, the subjects are first randomized either to a new treatment or a standard treatment. After being enrolled in one treatment (e.g., treatment A), patients are followed for a certain period of time and observed for changes in outcome. These patients are then switched over to the other treatment group (e.g., treatment B). Similarly, patients who received treatment B first are also switched over to treatment A after a certain period of observation and ascertainment of outcome. Both groups are then observed again for a certain period of time, and changes in outcome are measured (Figure 9.4).

Changes in outcome in patients when they were in treatment group A can be compared with the same patients when they were in treatment group B. Similarly, changes in outcome in patients when they were in treatment group B can be compared to when they were in treatment group A. Therefore, each patient serves as his or her own control. This design ensures that the intervention and control groups are comparable and thus prevents selection bias in the study.

Crossover designs have some drawbacks, such as: a) there may be a carry-over effect from the drug the subjects received in Period 1 (Figure 9.4). For example, if a subject is switched from treatment A (in Period 1) to treatment B (in Period 2) and observed under each treatment, the observation under

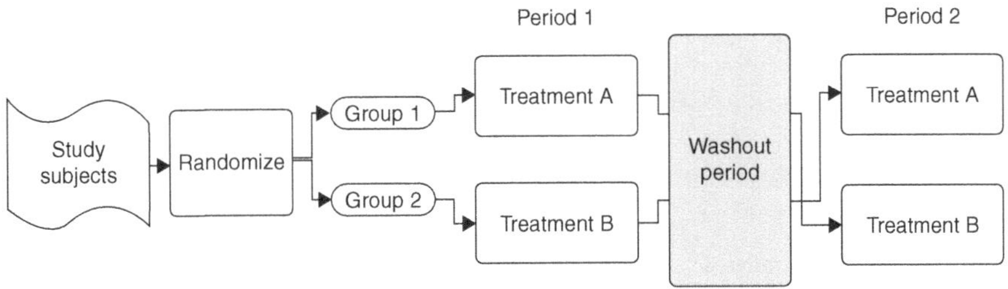

FIGURE 9.4

Crossover design.

treatment B may be affected by the residual effects of treatment A. Therefore, a washout period is needed to ensure that none of the effects of treatment A remain (Figure 9.4); b) a planned crossover trial is not possible for surgical interventions; c) if the new therapy cures the disease under investigation, crossover trial is not possible; d) patients may drop out after the first treatment; and e) the order in which treatments are given may illicit psychological effects, and the patients may react differently to the treatment given first.

Unplanned crossovers can occur in a parallel design of clinical trials. In an unplanned crossover trial, patients may be shifted from one treatment group to another if they change their minds. For example, a patient may decide to be treated with another regimen than the one s/he was assigned to, or if a patient in one group deteriorates during the trial, he or she may need to be shifted to the other group. As a result, some patients who were assigned to Treatment A may be shifted to Treatment B and vice versa, which breaks the benefits of randomization.

If the data are analyzed according to the original assignment (called an intention-to-treat [ITT] analysis), some patients who actually received treatment B will be included in treatment group A, and vice versa. On the other hand, if the data are analyzed according to the treatment actually received, excluding those who deviated and lost to follow-up (per-protocol analysis), randomization is broken, and the benefits of random allocation are lost. There is no perfect solution to this dilemma. The current recommendation is to use the ITT analysis. However, since there is no perfect solution to this problem, investigators should always try to keep the unplanned crossover to a minimum.

9.4.3 Factorial Design

A factorial design is not frequently used in clinical trials. In factorial designs, two treatments (e.g., treatments A and B) can be evaluated simultaneously with each other in a single study. In this design, patients are divided into four groups: a) patients who received only treatment A and B) patients who received only treatment B; c) patients who received both A and B; and d) patients who received a standard treatment or a placebo (Figure 9.5). This

		Treatment A	
		Yes	No
Treatment B	Yes	Both A & B	Only B
	No	Only A	Standard treatment or placebo

FIGURE 9.5

Factorial design in clinical trials.

design offers the opportunity for multiple comparisons, such as comparing the effects of treatment A against treatment B, evaluating the effect of treatment A or B against the standard treatment (or placebo), assessing the combined effect of treatments A and B against the standard treatment (or placebo), and examining the potential interactions between treatments A and B.

9.4.4 Pre-Post Design

In a pre-post or before-after design, the outcome indicator of the study group(s) is measured at the baseline and after the intervention. The post-intervention assessment may be a single measurement or multiple (repeated) measurements. A before-after study that includes only a single measurement of the outcome before and after the intervention has the highest risk of bias. Therefore, studies with multiple post-intervention measurements are more advantageous [5].

A pre-post design may or may not have a comparison group. When a study has one or more comparison groups, it is referred to as *controlled before-after design*. If the study does not have a comparison group (an uncontrolled trial), it is called a *quasi-experimental* design. A single group before-after design, compared to a randomized controlled trial, cannot provide definitive evidence that the differences seen in the outcome variable are because of the intervention. Changes in the outcome are unreliable and may be due to the placebo effect, lifestyle change, or other factors [6].

An example of a before-after clinical trial design with a comparison group and repeated measurements is a study in which a researcher evaluates the effectiveness of a new drug in reducing blood sugar levels in diabetic patients compared to a standard treatment (a pre-post controlled trial design). In this study, the researcher may be interested in measuring the blood sugar levels of study subjects at the baseline (before administration of the drugs under investigation) and two hours, six hours, and 12 hours after administration of the drugs in both groups. The data are then analyzed using relevant statistical methods. This design is similar to the parallel design.

A pre-post design with a single measurement of the outcome before and after the intervention is common in community trials [7, 8]. Community trials also frequently use cluster-randomized controlled pre-post designs to evaluate the effectiveness of interventions [9].

9.5 Blinding

Blinding, also known as masking, is a feature in clinical trial design that prevents investigators and/or participants from knowing which treatment has been assigned to each participant. In clinical trials, both patients and researchers can be blinded. When only the patients are unaware of the treatment they are receiving, it is called a single-blind trial. When neither patients nor investigators, including those who are involved in patient care and evaluation, know which treatment a patient is on, it is called a *double-blind* study. Blinding mostly prevents information bias in the study. The use of the single-blind method is particularly important when the outcome measure is subjective, such as pain (e.g., headache or joint pain).

   Blinding can be done by using a placebo. A placebo is an inert substance that looks, tests, and smells like the active drug used in the treatment group. The use of a placebo is particularly helpful when evaluating the frequency of side effects of a drug. However, the use of a placebo may not guarantee that the patients are masked. Some patients may guess whether they are taking a placebo or an active drug.

9.6 Selection of Subjects

Before organizing a clinical trial, patient entry requirements need to be carefully decided. A clear, specific, and objective case definition and eligibility criteria (including the exclusion criteria) in writing need to be developed to enroll patients in the study. The patients to be included in a study should represent the disease under investigation so that the trial's findings can be generalized (i.e., applied to the entire population of such patients). For example, if a clinical trial is planned for patients with asthma admitted to a hospital, these patients may represent only the severe cases rather than the typical cases of asthma. Therefore, the issue of representativeness needs careful attention. The principal aspects of patient selection include: a) the disease state under investigation (clear eligibility criteria); b) exclusion criteria; and c) the source of patient recruitment.

9.7 Control Group

A trial may not have a control group (see Section 9.4.4), such as a single-group pre-post design. Trials without a control group may provide initial insights about the efficacy of a drug for further investigation. Since improvement on an outcome with a treatment may be due to the placebo effect, a control group is needed for a trial to draw a causal inference about the relationship between a treatment and outcome. There are several options for selecting a control group, such as: a) historical or non-concurrent controls; b) concurrent nonrandomized controls; and c) concurrent randomized controls.

9.7.1 Historical Controls

When controls are selected from patients already treated in the past (before starting the trial), it is called the historical control. Historical controls are of value when the disease is highly fatal and there is a common understanding that the new treatment reduces the fatality rate significantly. For historical controls, information is obtained from patients' records with the same disease who were treated earlier with standard treatment. Data from historical controls are compared with those of patients receiving the new treatment in a prospective trial to conclude the results. For example, Ahmed et al. (1999) evaluated the effectiveness of a standardized management protocol (new treatment) for the reduction of mortality in severely malnourished children using a historical control [10]. In this study, the mortality rate of malnourished children treated with the standard protocol from January to June 1997 was compared with a group (historical control) treated during the same time period in 1996, before the standard protocol was implemented.

Although the use of a historical control group is attractive and less expensive, a major limitation is that the data from historical controls and their quality may not be comparable since the data were not recorded for the purpose of research. Data collected prospectively and for the purpose of research usually uses meticulous data collection methods. Other limitations include: a) there may be differences in patient selection criteria between two groups (historical controls are less likely to use clearly defined criteria for patient selection); b) the control group may not be comparable to patients in the new treatment group; and c) patient response criteria may differ between two groups. As a result, if a difference is observed in the new treatment outcome, it may be difficult to say whether or not the difference is due to the new treatment or because of differences in patient selection criteria or data quality.

9.7.2 Concurrent Nonrandomized Controls

Controls can be selected with or without a random selection process. In concurrent (simultaneous) nonrandomized controls, controls are selected without a random selection process. The use of nonrandomized controls severely reduces the credibility of study results. One approach to selecting the nonrandomized controls is to select patients based on the day of the month or by alternating patients in the treatment groups, a method known as systematic allocation (see Section 9.8.1). For instance, it may be decided that patients selected on odd-numbered days will receive the new treatment, while patients selected on even-numbered days will receive the standard treatment (or placebo). The problem with this selection method is that the investigator can predict in advance the treatment the next patient will receive. Such prior knowledge about treatment allocation may influence patient selection into the treatment groups, leading to bias.

9.7.3 Concurrent Randomized Controls

In concurrent randomized controls, controls are selected using a random selection process, such as randomization (Section 9.8). Simultaneous selection of randomized controls, where the investigator does not know what treatment the next patient will receive, is the best and most efficient option for selecting controls and should be preferred in all clinical trials.

9.8 Treatment Allocation: Randomization

Treatment can be assigned to patients in a clinical trial through a random (randomized trial) or nonrandom (nonrandomized trial) process. Nonrandomized trials are called *quasi-experimental designs*. Randomization is the most commonly used method to decide which treatment each patient will receive in the trial. In randomized trials, study subjects are assigned either to receive an intervention (e.g., a new treatment) or a standard treatment (or a placebo) using a random process. When treatment is assigned through a random process, the trial is called a randomized trial. Randomization gives patients equal chances of receiving either treatment. It is therefore an unbiased method of allocating treatment to study participants.

The main purpose of randomization is to prevent selection bias that might be introduced by investigators in assigning participants to treatment groups, i.e., the process of randomization removes the control of investigators in deciding treatment assignments. Randomization usually ensures that study groups are comparable in terms of known and unknown factors, especially when the sample size is large, though it does not guarantee that the treatment groups will be similar. A randomized double-blind controlled trial is acknowledged as the "gold standard" in the evaluation of the efficacy of a new treatment. Randomization is done before patients are assigned to treatment groups (Figure 9.2) in the study. There are several ways of allocating treatments to patients, as discussed below.

9.8.1 Systematic Assignments

In clinical trials, patients are sometimes assigned to various treatment groups using predetermined systematic methods, such as: a) assigning treatment based on the date of birth (e.g., if the date of birth falls on an even day, the patient will receive the new treatment; if on an odd day, the patient will receive the standard treatment or a placebo); b) assigning treatment according to the date of presentation or admission (e.g., patients presenting on even days will receive the new treatment, while those presenting on odd days will receive the standard treatment or a placebo); or c) using alternate assignment (e.g., patients with odd registration numbers will receive the new treatment, while patients with even registration numbers will receive the standard treatment or a placebo). The main issue with these methods is that the investigator can easily predict which treatment the next patient will receive if they are enrolled in the study. This prior knowledge may influence the investigator's decision regarding a patient's entry into the trial, leading to selection bias and thus affecting the validity of the results.

Another method of assignment that is also occasionally used is *judgment assignment*. In this approach, investigators decide which treatment to assign from several options based on their own judgment. This method can introduce significant bias into the study, as the investigator might favor assigning a particular treatment to less serious patients, leading to better outcomes regardless of the treatment's actual benefit. Therefore, judgmental assignment is generally regarded as unacceptable in clinical trials.

9.8.2 Simple Randomization

For the random assignment of treatments using simple randomization, a randomization list is first prepared either by using a random number table or computer-generated random numbers. Suppose that a randomized trial has two groups – one group will receive drug A, and the other group will receive drug B. Let us decide that if the random number digit is zero to four, treatment A will be assigned, and if the random number digit is five to nine, treatment B will be assigned. Now, generate the random numbers using the computer (or the random number table). Suppose that the computer has generated the random numbers as shown in Table 9.1. The sequence of treatments the patients will receive is, therefore, A B B A B B A B A.

For a trial involving three groups (e.g., treatments A, B, and C), one may decide that if:

- Random number digit is one to three, assign treatment A;
- Random number digit is four to six, assign treatment B;

TABLE 9.1

Simple randomization method

Random numbers	2	7	6	0	5	8	3	9	1
Treatment allocation	A	B	B	A	B	B	A	B	A

- Random number digit is seven to nine, assign treatment C; and
- Ignore if the random digit is zero.

You can make the randomization list as long as it is needed. The disadvantage of the simple randomization method is that the treatment groups may end up with unequal sizes, especially when the sample size is small.

The randomization list for the allocation of treatment should be prepared by an independent person (e.g., a doctor, nurse, or statistician not involved in the study). The types of treatment (as per the randomization list) can be written on cards and put into sealed envelopes sequentially. The investigating clinician or nurse can open the envelope sequentially and assign the treatment upon enrollment of each patient. If the trial is double-blinded, the pharmacist involved in the trial can prepare the drugs. In that case, he or she needs to be given the randomization list beforehand to prepare the drug packages, which should be identical in appearance.

9.8.3 Random Permuted Blocks

This method ensures an equal number of patients in each treatment group. For a two-treatment trial (e.g., drug A and drug B), blocks are prepared as AB and BA. Based on the random number digits, either treatment A or treatment B is assigned.

For instance, let us decide that the treatment sequence will be AB if the random digit is zero to four, while the treatment sequence will be BA if the random digit is five to nine. The following table (Table 9.2) shows the random numbers generated by a computer and the corresponding allocation of treatment.

Therefore, prepare the randomization list for the treatment allocation, starting with A B B A …, i.e., the enrolled patients will receive treatment in the sequence of A B B A…

9.8.4 Stratified Randomization

In stratified randomization, enrolled patients are first stratified (categorized) into groups based on selected characteristics. Then, either simple randomization or the permuted random block method is applied to generate a separate randomization list for each stratum. For instance, a researcher might use stratified randomization to balance groups by the status of diabetes (present

TABLE 9.2

Permuted random block method of randomization

Random numbers	2	7	6	0	5	8	3	9	1
Treatment allocation	AB	BA	BA	AB	BA	BA	AB	BA	AB

or absent) when diabetes is considered a strong confounding or prognostic factor for the study outcome.

9.9 Treatment Schedule and Compliance

Clinical trials are mainly focused on the evaluation of drug therapy. Clinical trials can also be conducted for the evaluation of non-drug therapies, such as surgical procedures, dietary interventions, hospital care versus home care, or other types of interventions. When a clinical trial is planned to evaluate a drug therapy, the features that need to be carefully considered include a) dose, b) frequency of administration, c) route of administration, and d) duration of therapy [2].

Occasionally, it may require an adjustment of the dose to minimize the side effects. As such, guidelines should be developed in the planning phase to decide on dose modification or withdrawal of a drug. Supportive (ancillary) treatments may also be required while managing patients. The investigators need to specify what non-protocol drugs for ancillary care are permissible and under what circumstances. Such ancillary care should be used consistently in both treatment groups [2, 11].

In order to protect the welfare of patients, a decision needs to be made on the early termination of the trial before it is originally scheduled. In such cases, interim analyses by an independent group are planned. If the data indicate clear benefits on the primary outcome of interest or if one treatment is clearly harmful, then early termination of the trial should be considered. However, a decision on early termination depends on several other factors and should be considered with great caution [11].

For example, White et al. (1989) conducted a clinical trial to evaluate the efficacy of ceftazidime against the standard therapy in reducing mortality in patients with severe melioidosis [12]. Melioidosis causes severe illness and has a high case fatality rate (about 80%). In the planning phase of the trial, it was decided to reduce the dose of ceftazidime for patients who would develop renal failure and to change the treatment regimen to the other group if there was no evidence of clinical response after six days of treatment. The trial was stopped before the scheduled time when a significant reduction in mortality in the treatment group of ceftazidime was achieved to protect the welfare of patients.

Patients' compliance with therapy is an important concern. It is common to observe that some patients do not comply with the treatment schedule. Noncompliance reduces the trial's ability to detect differences in treatment effects. Noncompliance is particularly common among outpatients treated with repeated doses of oral drugs administered by the patients themselves.

In clinical trials, patients' compliance with treatment needs to be closely monitored. Compliance should be checked during regular follow-up visits. Patients should be asked to bring unused pills with them during all follow-up visits, and compliance can be checked simply by counting the number of unused pills. If there are more or fewer unused pills than expected (based on the intended dose schedule), this is a clear indication of noncompliance. However, if the pill count is correct, it does not guarantee that compliance is ensured. Compliance can also be assessed based on the self-report of patients, particularly in non-drug intervention trials (e.g., the effect of exercise or a dietary regimen on an outcome of interest). In some instances, compliance is checked by blood or urine tests through drug assays.

It is important to identify the reasons for noncompliance. Noncompliance can be due to side effects of a drug, a lack of patients' cooperation, misunderstandings, or an inconvenient drug schedule (e.g., a drug therapy every four hours). Careful counseling on the importance of taking drugs as per schedule with an explanation of the trial's objective, labeling of the dose schedule on the drugs provided, and frequent contact with patients over telephone, e-mail, or other means are helpful in minimizing noncompliance. For a long-duration trial, scheduling a long follow-up period may increase the risk of non-compliance. The follow-up schedule should therefore be carefully planned (follow-up visits every two to four weeks may be a suitable choice).

9.10 Protocol Deviations

A protocol deviation is any intentional or unintentional departure from the study design, treatment plan, or study procedures specified in the study protocol approved by the institutional review board (IRB). A protocol deviation occurs when a researcher does not fully adhere to the IRB-approved protocol, or when study subjects fail to adhere to the treatment protocol. Depending on the severity, protocol deviations may place participants at risk and can compromise the scientific integrity of the study, thus jeopardizing the justification for the research.

The problem of protocol deviation may vary from patients' withdrawal from the treatment to minor lapses in the treatment or evaluation schedule. Minor deviations are almost inevitable in clinical trials. Examples of protocol deviations include: a) enrolling an ineligible participant; b) failing to obtain informed consent before enrolling a participant; c) performing a study procedure not approved by the IRB; d) omitting a required lab test; e) making dosing errors in study medication; and f) allowing an unauthorized person to evaluate a participant.

The aim of a clinical trial should be to follow the approved protocol strictly, identify all protocol deviations early (along with their reasons), and minimize the risk of future deviations as much as possible. Based on their impact, protocol deviations can be categorized as follows [2]:

Protocol violations: Protocol violations are serious deviations from the approved study protocol that can impact the safety, rights, or well-being of study subjects and could have been prevented by the investigators. Such violations can also affect the accuracy, completeness, or reliability of study data, thereby compromising the study's results. Examples of protocol violations include enrolling an ineligible participant, failing to obtain informed consent, or performing a study procedure not approved by the IRB.

Major deviations: Major deviations are departures from the approved study protocol that could impact the safety of study participants and the integrity of data, often arising from factors beyond the control of the research team. Such deviations may result from actions taken by study subjects or the research team. Examples include non-adherence to treatment by study subjects, a participant's refusal to complete scheduled activities, or an unintentional change or non-compliance with the research protocol (e.g., due to an unexpected adverse effect of a drug requiring protocol adjustment). Other examples are unexpected comorbidities (e.g., the occurrence of an acute attack of asthma in a patient) necessitating immediate treatment or technological failures (e.g., a malfunction of an electronic monitoring device).

Minor deviations: A minor protocol deviation is any change or departure from the study design or procedures in an approved research protocol that is unlikely to impact the subject's rights, safety, health, or well-being, or the completeness, accuracy, and reliability of study data. Examples include a participant missing a scheduled visit, a rescheduled study visit, or a required lab test not being performed when it does not affect the subject's safety or the study results.

Protocol violations and major deviations must be reported promptly to the IRB, along with a risk assessment detailing how these changes may affect the integrity and validity of the study. Minor protocol deviations are recorded and typically reported at the next review meeting. Investigators can maintain a deviation log to document minor deviations and report it for review at scheduled review meetings.

9.11 Patient Evaluation

For a reliable evaluation of the efficacy of an intervention, data collection from all groups should be of the same quality. Attention must be given to ensure comparable data collection from all subjects, irrespective of the treatment groups to avoid information bias. It is not desirable to have differences in results due to differences in the quality of data collection.

Data related to prognostic factors should also be collected from all participants at baseline (i.e., on entry to the study). The baseline characteristics are compared between groups to check whether they are comparable, even though randomization is done. Data on which treatment the patient was assigned to and which treatment the patient actually received needs to be collected. Compliance with the treatment schedule is also important to note.

A complete measurement of the outcome variable(s) in all study subjects needs to be ascertained. The outcome measures should include both improvements and side effects that have occurred. The measurement of outcomes must be based on explicit and predefined criteria. The outcome measures should be evaluated using the same quality instrument in both groups.

9.12 Sample Size

How many subjects are needed for a clinical trial should be decided in the planning phase. The sample size should be sufficiently large to protect a trial from two types of errors. One is the *Type I error (α)*, which indicates the probability of rejecting the null hypothesis when there is actually no association between treatment and outcome. The other one is the *Type II error (β)*, which indicates the probability of not rejecting the null hypothesis when there is actually an association between treatment and outcome. The quantity of one minus β ($1 - \beta$) is called the *power* of the study (also see Section 17.2.1). To calculate the sample size for a clinical trial, the following key questions need to be answered [2]:

- What is the main purpose of the study?
- What is the principal measure of patient outcome? How will the data be analyzed to determine the treatment difference, and at what level of significance (α)?
- What type of results does one anticipate with the standard treatment (i.e., what proportion of patients develop the outcome in the standard treatment group)?
- How small a treatment difference is important to detect, and with what degree of certainty (power of the study)?

With all the information and using the formula as presented in Section 17.5, one can easily calculate the sample size for a clinical trial.

9.13 Statistical Analyses

The method of statistical analysis of data depends on the study objectives and outcome measures. It is valuable to specify the statistical analysis plan before the trial starts. One should not be too inflexible about the use of statistical methods for data analysis, as planned at the beginning. However, a little modification may be needed depending on the situation.

The basic approach to the data analysis of a clinical trial is similar to the data analysis of a cohort study, as discussed in Chapter 8. Like cohort studies, rates of outcome in intervention and control groups are compared in clinical trials. The role of bias, chance, and confounding factors needs to be carefully evaluated before concluding the results.

Relevant basic characteristics of study subjects in treatment and comparison groups must be compared at the beginning to demonstrate that balance is achieved in the groups, and should be presented first in the results section of the report. If there is an imbalance in such characteristics between groups, especially the confounding factors, data need to be adjusted during analysis using relevant multivariable statistical techniques (e.g., logistic regression, multiple linear regression, or Cox regression, depending on the nature of the outcome variable and objective of the trial) [2, 13, 14].

Another important issue is deciding whether patients who did not comply with the treatment schedule, patients with protocol deviations, and withdrawals should be included in the analysis. Some investigators exclude these cases from analysis (per-protocol analysis). Exclusion of any randomized patients from analysis leads to biased results. Therefore, in all circumstances, data should be analyzed using the intention-to-treat (ITT) approach [6, 15]. The ITT analysis includes all patients randomly allocated to groups. The analysis is based on the initial treatment assignment and not on the treatment actually received. The ITT analysis ignores noncompliance, protocol deviations, withdrawal, and anything else that happens after randomization [15]. This approach to data analysis maintains the prognostic balance generated from the original random allocation.

Since problems like noncompliance, withdrawal, and protocol deviations are common in clinical trials, the aim of all trials should be to achieve a high level of compliance, keep losses to follow-up to a minimum, and collect complete information on all randomized patients.

References

1. Friedman LM, Furberg CD, DeMets DL, Reboussin DM, Granger CB. *Fundamentals of Clinical Trials*. 5th ed. Switzerland: Springer; 2015.

2.   Pocock JS. *Clinical Trials: A Practical Approach.* New York: Wiley; 1984.
3.   Gordis L. *Epidemiology.* 5th ed. Philadelphia: Elsevier Saunders; 2014.
4.   Altman DG. *Practical Statistics for Medical Research.* 1st ed. New York: Chapman & Hill; 1992.
5.   Ma S, Wang T. The optimal pre-post allocation for randomized clinical trials. *BMC Med Res Methodol.* 2023;23:72.
6.   Aggarwal R, Ranganathan P. Study designs: Part 4 – Interventional studies. *Perspect Clin Res.* 2019;10(3):137–9.
7.   Yang Y, Dai J, Min J, Song Z, Zha S, Chang L, et al. Evaluation of stroke health education for primary school students in Dali, China. *Front Public Health.* 2022;10:861792. doi:10.3389/fpubh.2022.861792
8.   Jacobs C, Michelo C, Chola M, Oliphant N, Halwiindi H, Maswenyeho S, et al. Evaluation of a community-based intervention to improve maternal and neonatal health service coverage in the most rural and remote districts of Zambia. *PLoS ONE.* 2018;13(1):e0190145. doi:10.1371/journal.pone.0190145
9.   Azad K, Barnett S, Banerjee B, Shaha S, Khan K, Rego AR, et al. Effect of scaling up women's groups on birth outcomes in three rural districts in Bangladesh: A cluster-randomized controlled trial. *Lancet.* 2010;375(9721):1193–202. doi:10.1016/S0140-6736(10)60142-0
10. Ahmed T, Ali M, Ullah MM, Choudhury IA, Haque ME, Salam MA, et al. Mortality in severely malnourished children with diarrhea and use of a standardized management protocol. *Lancet.* 1999;353:1919–22. doi:10.1016/S0140-6736(98)07499-6
11. Hennekens CH, Buring JE. *Epidemiology in Medicine.* Boston/Toronto: Little Brown and Company; 1987.
12. White NJ, Dance DAB, Chaowagul W, Wattanagoon Y, Wuthiekanun V, Pitakwatchara N. Halving of mortality of severe melioidosis by ceftazidime. *Lancet.* 1989;2(8665):697–701. doi:10.1016/S0140-6736(89)90768-X
13. Islam MT, Kabir R, Nisha M. *Data Analysis with Stata: A Comprehensive Guide for Data Analysis and Interpretation of Outputs.* Dhaka, Bangladesh: ASA Publications; 2022.
14. Islam MT, Kabir R, Nisha M. *Learning SPSS without Pain.* 2nd ed. Dhaka, Bangladesh: ASA Publications; 2021.
15. Gupta SK. Intention-to-treat concept: A review. *Perspect Clin Res.* 2011;2(3):109–12. doi:10.4103/2229-3485.83221

10

Survival Analysis

Mohammad Tajul Islam

In epidemiology, survival analysis is a popular data analysis approach for certain kinds of data. In general, survival analysis is a collection of statistical procedures for data analysis for which the outcome variable is the time until an event occurs. In most clinical studies, the outcome of interest is death, and data are available on the time taken for an event to occur. Survival analysis methods are particularly employed to analyze the time-to-event data collected from cohort studies or clinical trials [1–6].

In cohort studies and clinical trials, it is nearly always not possible to follow all subjects for exactly the same length of time because individuals are recruited at different time points and may also leave the study at different times. Another difficulty in such studies is that the exact survival times (i.e., lengths of time from enrollment in a study to the development of outcome) are only known for those who experience the outcome of interest, while the survival times remain unknown for others (e.g., who are lost to follow-up and do not develop the outcome during the study period) in the study group [4].

Death is commonly considered the outcome of interest in many studies. However, the outcome of interest can be other measures, such as recurrence of a disease (e.g., cancer), appearance of a symptom, recovery from a condition (e.g., coma), or discharge from the hospital. In survival analysis, it is important to note the outcome of interest and the period of observation until the occurrence of the outcome or loss from the study.

Survival analysis answers two basic questions that are of considerable interest to both clinicians and patients. They are: a) what is the average survival time (the median survival time), and b) what is the probability that a patient with a disease (or on a treatment) will survive for a specified duration of time from a given point in time until the occurrence of an outcome, such as death, recurrence of a disease, or others [3, 4]?

In Chapter 3, the basic concepts of survival analysis, such as the life table approach and the Kaplan-Meier method, have been discussed. This chapter discusses how to compare the survival probabilities in two groups of individuals,

DOI: 10.1201/9781003654803-10

including how to produce and interpret the survival curve, calculate the median survival time, and test survival differences between two groups.

10.1 Survival Time

Suppose a researcher is interested in evaluating the effectiveness of a new drug (e.g., drug B) compared to the standard drug (e.g., drug A) in preventing a second heart attack (myocardial infarction or MI) over a five-year period following an initial heart attack (MI). To conduct the study, the researcher enrolled some MI patients and randomly assigned them to receive either drug A or drug B. Each patient enrolled in the study was followed during the study period, and their outcomes were recorded. In a study like this, enrolled patients will experience one of the following three outcomes during the study period:

- Develop a second MI (outcome of interest);
- Lost to follow-up for reasons such as migration, death from causes other than MI, or other reasons; or
- Remain free from a second attack of MI until the end of the study.

One important measure to record in such studies is the length of time (in terms of days, weeks, months, or years) that each patient elapsed between the point of enrollment and the occurrence of any of the above outcomes. The length of time that each patient elapses between the enrollment point and one of the above outcomes is called the *survival time*. The dataset containing the survival times of study subjects is called the *survival data*.

Survival time is of two types: *event time and censored time*. Event time is the time contributed by study subjects who develop the outcome of interest (the event), while censored time is the time contributed by study subjects who are lost to follow-up or subjects who survive (do not develop the outcome) until the end of the study period.

In connection with the above example, suppose we have the following information on three patients enrolled in the study. The outcome of interest is the development of a second MI.

- *Patient A:* Enrolled in the study on 1 January 2015 and developed the second MI (the event) on 31 July of the same year;
- *Patient B:* Enrolled in the study on 1 March 2015 and was lost to follow-up after moving out of the city on 30 April 2016; and
- *Patient C:* Entered the study on 1 August 2015 and did not develop a second MI (did not develop the event) by the termination of the study on 31 December 2019.

Patient B was lost from the study after 14 months of follow-up. The amount of survival time contributed by patient B to the study is therefore 14 months, which is the *censored survival time* (since the patient did not develop the outcome). Similarly, for patient C, who remained in the study until the end of the study period, the survival time (53 months) is also considered a censored survival time. Thus, the survival times for patients B and C are considered *censored data*. On the other hand, the seven-month time that patient A has elapsed from enrollment to the development of a second MI (the event of interest) is the *event time*. In survival analysis, both event time and censored time (together called survival time) are used to analyze the data.

10.2 Comparison of Survival Experiences

Survival analysis can be employed to compare the survival experiences of two or more groups of patients. In studies where two treatment groups are compared, the researcher is interested in three types of information from each enrolled patient. They are:

- Which treatment did the patient receive (e.g., drug A or B)?
- For what length of time was the patient observed (length of observation)?
- Did the patient experience the event of interest (in our example, a second attack of MI) during the study period, or was the patient either lost to follow-up or alive without developing a second MI until the end of the study (i.e., whether the observed time is event time or censored time)?

With this information, it is possible to estimate the median survival times for both groups for comparison. Such a comparison allows us to answer the question: "Which treatment increases or delays time to the occurrence of the event of interest (i.e., the second attack of MI)"? Additionally, data collected in a follow-up study can answer another important question: "What is the estimated probability that a patient will survive for a specified length of time"? For example, what is the probability that a patient with a first MI, receiving treatment A (or B), will survive (i.e., will not develop a second MI) for more than five years?

Methods applied to answer these questions in a follow-up study are known as survival analysis methods. Survival analyses can be done using either the classic life table approach or the Kaplan-Meier procedure. The Kaplan-Meier procedure is more efficient and is the most frequently used method for survival data analysis. Here, the Kaplan-Meier method is used to analyze the data of the following example.

Example
Suppose that a researcher conducted a clinical trial to evaluate the effectiveness of a new drug (drug B) for the prevention of death (outcome of interest)

due to an acute heart attack (MI) compared to the standard treatment (drug A) over a period of six months. To conduct the study, 44 MI patients were recruited and randomly assigned to either drug A (n=22) or drug B (n=22). Survival data (hypothetical) of this study is presented in Table 10.1. Survival analysis can be done using computer data analysis software, such as SPSS, Stata, R, or SAS. Stata software was used to analyze the data [7], and the results are presented in Tables 10.2 to 10.5 and Figure 10.1.

TABLE 10.1

Survival data of 44 patients with an acute heart attack

Treatment group: A			Treatment group: B		
Patient no.	Survival time (days)	Outcome: 1= died 0= censored	Patient no.	Survival time (days)	Outcome: 1= died 0= censored
1	2	1	23	2	1
2	3	1	24	6	1
3	4	1	25	12	1
4	7	1	26	54	1
5	10	1	27	56	0
6	22	1	28	68	1
7	28	1	29	89	1
8	29	1	30	96	1
9	32	1	31	96	1
10	37	1	32	125	0
11	40	1	33	128	0
12	41	1	34	131	0
13	54	1	35	140	0
14	61	1	36	141	0
15	63	1	37	143	1
16	71	1	38	145	0
17	127	0	39	146	1
18	140	0	40	148	0
19	146	0	41	59	1
20	158	0	42	60	1
21	167	0	43	44	0
22	182	0	44	60	0

Table 10.2 shows the number of study subjects and deaths that occurred in the treatment groups. In total, 44 patients were enrolled in this study, of whom 22 received drug A and another 22 received drug B. The table shows that there were more deaths in the treatment group A [16 out of 22 (72.7%)] compared to the treatment group B [11 out of 22 (50.0%)]. This may indicate a better probability of survival for patients in treatment group B.

10.2.1 Median Survival Time

The median survival time is the length of time when the cumulative survival probability is 0.50, i.e., the time when 50% of the subjects develop the event. In survival analyses, the median is preferred over the mean because the median is not affected by extreme values (outliers). On the other hand, to calculate the mean survival time, it is required to observe the event (outcome of interest) for all study subjects, which is not realistic.

Table 10.3 shows the median survival times (under column 50%) for both treatment groups, including their 95% confidence intervals (CIs). The median survival time can also be estimated by locating the time point at which the

TABLE 10.2

Survival status of study subjects

```
Treatment |    Survival status
    group | Censored        Died |     Total
----------+---------------------+----------
   drug A |        6          16 |        22
          |    27.27       72.73 |    100.00
----------+---------------------+----------
   drug B |       11          11 |        22
          |    50.00       50.00 |    100.00
----------+---------------------+----------
    Total |       17          27 |        44
          |    38.64       61.36 |    100.00
```

TABLE 10.3

Median survival time with 95% confidence interval (50% is the median survival time)

```
. stci, by(treatment)
              |     no. of
  treatment   |   subjects     50%    Std. Err.    [95% Conf. Interval]
--------------+-----------------------------------------------------------
       drug A |       22        40    12.89864      22               71
       drug B |       22       146    10.79461      89                .
--------------+-----------------------------------------------------------
        total |       44        89    21.23218      41              168
```

cumulative survival proportion equals 0.50 in the survival table or on the survival curve. The table shows that the median survival time for patients who received drug A is 40 days (95% CI: 22 – 71), while it is 146 days (95% CI: 89 – .) for those who received drug B. This indicates that drug B increases the survival time more than that of drug A (i.e., drug B is associated with a longer time-to-event compared to drug A).

10.2.2 Survival Probability for Two Groups

A comparison of survival functions (cumulative survival probabilities) at different time points for the treatment groups is provided in Table 10.4. For instance, at 46 days, the cumulative survival probability is 0.45 (45%) in treatment group A, while it is 0.86 (86%) in treatment group B. The cumulative survival probabilities are also consistently higher in treatment group B than in treatment group A at time points from 68 days to 156 days. This indicates a higher probability of survival if a patient is in treatment group B than in treatment group A. In other words, it suggests the benefits of drug B.

However, if we consider the cumulative survival probability of patients in both groups at the end of the study period (178 days), the survival probabilities are not that different (0.272 in the treatment group A and 0.304 in the treatment group B). This information suggests that though survival experiences are significantly different between the treatment groups (as indicated by the log-rank test; Table 10.5), the difference in survival probability at the end of the study (six months) is very small.

Now, the question is whether the survival experiences of both of these groups in the population are different or not. For an objective comparison of survival experiences in two groups, it is desirable to use a statistical method

TABLE 10.4

Comparison of survival status

```
. sts list, by (treatment) compare
                            Survivor           Function
          treatment          drug A             drug B
          -----------------------------------------------
          time          2     0.9545             0.9545
                       24     0.7273             0.8636
                       46     0.4545             0.8636
                       68     0.3182             0.7701
                       90     0.2727             0.7219
                      112     0.2727             0.6257
                      134     0.2727             0.6257
                      156     0.2727             0.4562
                      178     0.2727             0.3041
          -----------------------------------------------
```

TABLE 10.5

Log-rank test

```
. sts test treatment
Log-rank test for equality of survivor functions
              |        Events         Events
treatment     |      observed       expected
--------------+-------------------------------
drug A        |            16          10.62
drug B        |            11          16.38
--------------+-------------------------------
Total         |            27          27.00

                      chi2(1) =          4.66
                      Pr>chi2 =        0.0309
```

that will tell us whether the difference in survival experiences in the population is statistically significant or not. The commonly used statistical test to compare the survival experiences of two or more groups is the log-rank test.

10.2.3 Log-Rank Test

The log-rank test is used to determine whether the survival of study subjects in two or more groups is significantly different. Here, the null hypothesis is "there is no difference in the survival experience of subjects in treatment group A and treatment group B in the population". The log-rank test is an extension of the Mantel-Haenszel (MH) procedure applied after stratification of survival data.

Table 10.5 shows the results of the log-rank test. The p-value (Pr>chi2) of the test is 0.030 (less than 0.05), which is statistically significant at the 95% confidence level. This indicates that the survival experiences of the two groups in the population are not the same. In other words, it tells us that the probability of survival is higher (since the median survival time is higher in treatment group B) if a patient is in treatment group B than in treatment group A, i.e., drug B is more effective than drug A in increasing the survival probability.

There are alternative procedures for testing the null hypothesis that the two survival curves are identical. They are the Breslow test, the Tarone-Ware test, and the Peto test. The log-rank test ranks all the events (deaths in our example) equally, while the alternative tests give more weight to early events.

10.2.4 Survival Curve

The cumulative survival probability is commonly displayed through a graph called the survival curve. The steps in the graph represent the times when events (such as deaths or any other event of interest) occur. The graph allows us to visually compare the median survival times and cumulative survival probabilities of two or more groups over any specified time period.

Figure 10.1 illustrates the six-month survival curves of patients in two treatment groups: patients in treatment group A and patients in treatment group B. Six-month survival is the percentage of patients who are alive six months after initiation of the treatment. In this figure, the upper line represents the survival curve for patients who received treatment B. In general, the line above indicates a better survival probability.

In this example, the data show that survival rates at the end of six months are very similar in the two groups (27% in treatment group A and 30% in treatment group B; Table 10.4 and Figure 10.1). However, the survival curves for these two groups are different. Patients in group B experienced fewer deaths until about 60 days, whereas all deaths in treatment group A occurred within the first 70 days. Thus, even though the six-month survival rates are nearly identical in the two groups, survival during the six-month period was clearly better for patients in treatment group B compared to those in treatment group A.

Finally, survival analysis using the Kaplan-Meier method is based on certain assumptions, which include a) censoring of study participants is unrelated to the outcome, meaning the Kaplan-Meier method assumes that the

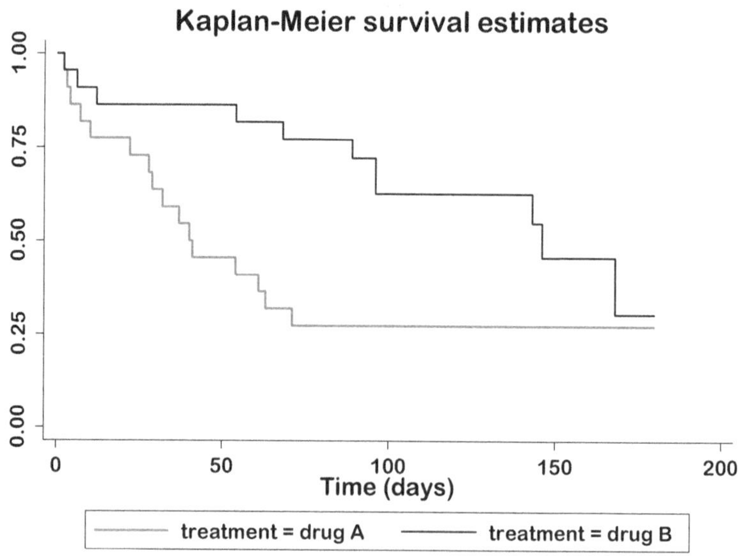

FIGURE 10.1
Survival curve.

probability of censoring is not related to the outcome of interest; b) survival probabilities are the same for participants recruited early and late in the study; and c) events occurred at the specified times [8].

References

1. Altman DG. *Practical Statistics for Medical Research.* 1st ed. New York: Chapman & Hall; 1992.
2. Chan YH. Biostatistics 203. Survival analysis. *Singapore Med J.* 2004;45(6):249–56.
3. Daniel WW. *Biostatistics: A Foundation for Analysis in the Health Sciences.* 7th ed. India: Wiley; 1999.
4. Gordis L. *Epidemiology.* 5th ed. Philadelphia: Elsevier Saunders; 2014.
5. Szklo M, Nieto FJ. *Epidemiology: Beyond the Basics.* 2nd ed. Boston: Jones and Bartlett Publishers; 2007.
6. Clark TG, Bradburn MJ, Love SB, Altman DG. Survival analysis part I: Basic concepts and first analyses. *Br J Cancer.* 2003;89(2):232–8. doi:10.1038/sj.bjc.6601118
7. Islam MT, Kabir R, Nisha M. *Data Analysis with Stata: A Comprehensive Guide for Data Analysis and Interpretation of Outputs.* 1st ed. Dhaka, Bangladesh: Altaf Publications; 2022.
8. Koletsi D, Pandis N. Survival analysis, part 2: Kaplan-Meier method and the log-rank test. *Am J Orthod Dentofacial Orthop.* 2017;152(4):569–71.

11

Evaluation of a Diagnostic Test and Screening in Health

Mohammad Tajul Islam

Practicing clinicians need to confirm the diagnosis of a disease for appropriate treatment. To arrive at a diagnosis, clinicians use various diagnostic tests to decide on a treatment plan. It is, therefore, important that clinicians understand the basic principles of diagnostic tests to interpret test results accurately.

On the other hand, the primary objective of public health is the prevention of diseases. Early detection and appropriate treatment are important strategies for disease prevention. The patterns of diseases seen at health facilities differ from those in the community. Diseases (e.g., diabetes, hypertension, or tuberculosis) that we observe at health facilities usually represent only a small portion of the diseases present in the community. The unrecognized diseases in the community may be subclinical cases, mild cases, carriers, or undiagnosed cases. For the purpose of prevention, it is important to detect unrecognized diseases in the community and bring them under treatment through screening for a better prognosis. This chapter discusses the basic principles of a diagnostic (or screening) test and the issues to consider when planning to detect unrecognized diseases in the general population through screening.

11.1 Evaluation of Screening or Diagnostic Tests

Whenever we plan for a screening program or aim to diagnose a disease, it is necessary to select and apply one or more tests initially to separate out individuals who may have the disease for further investigation to confirm the diagnosis. Various types of tests are available to differentiate healthy individuals from those who are sick.

Evaluation of a screening or diagnostic test is necessary before it is implemented in practice, when it is a new test or when selecting a test for

DOI: 10.1201/9781003654803-11

a screening program (or diagnosis) whose performance in detecting a disease is unknown. The primary objective of evaluating a test is to describe its ability to identify individuals who actually have the disease (or do not have the disease) of interest. Conventionally, when we refer to a test, we mean a laboratory test, such as a blood test, an X-ray, or other tests. However, a screening test may simply be a question, symptom, or sign. For example, in tuberculosis screening programs, the first screening test to identify individuals before a sputum test for acid-fast bacilli (AFB) is a question: "Do you have a cough for more than two weeks?" Whatever the nature of the test may be, it has two quantities to evaluate before it is used for the purpose of screening or diagnosis. They are *precision* and *validity*.

11.1.1 Precision

Precision is also called *repeatability or reliability*. Precision is the ability of a test to give consistent results on repeated applications. The precision of a test refers to how consistent and reproducible the test results are when it is repeated on the same individual or sample. When a test is precise, it demonstrates minimal random variation in its results. The precision of a test is examined on the same person under the same conditions. There are four sources of variability that can affect the precision of a test. Factors that may affect precision include [1, 2]:

> *Biological variation within individuals:* There are several characteristics of an individual that vary with time and other circumstances, even within the same individual. For example, the blood pressure of an individual. The blood pressure of an individual usually fluctuates with time (called diurnal variation) and other circumstances. The blood pressure may be different when measured in the morning than in the evening. Such a variation is not due to the instrument. It is because of the inherent characteristics of the factor being measured.

> *Variation due to test method and instrument (tool):* Precision may vary due to the test method and the instruments used to measure the same parameter. For example, variations in blood pressure may be observed if it is measured in a sitting position and in a lying position (variation due to the test method). Similarly, variations in blood hemoglobin levels may be present if they are measured by two different instruments (e.g., by a strip and by a hemocytometer) on the same individual (variation due to the instrument or tool).

> *Interobserver variation:* Interobserver variation refers to variations in measurements on the same subject by different evaluators (assessors). For example, if the blood pressure is measured by two or more individuals (assessors) on the same subject and using the same instrument, the measurements may be different. Another example is that if an X-ray

plate is given to two or more radiologists, the observations may not be the same.

Intraobserver variation: Intraobserver variation refers to variations in repeated measurements made by the same individual. For example, if the same X-ray plate is given to a radiologist on two or more occasions for reporting, the reports may differ.

Therefore, when evaluating the precision of a test, it is important to be aware of these factors. The influence of the above factors can be minimized by using a standard protocol for measurement, using the same instrument for all individuals, and providing training to the individuals involved in the measurement.

11.1.2 Validity

Validity is the ability of a test (or an instrument) to give the true value. It can be evaluated only if there is an accepted and independent method (the gold standard) to confirm the condition. There are two measures of validity, namely *sensitivity* and *specificity*. To determine the sensitivity and specificity of a test, it is necessary to apply the test to a group of individuals who have the disease and to another group of individuals who do not have the disease [2–9].

11.1.2.1 Sensitivity and Specificity

Sensitivity is the ability of a test to correctly classify individuals with the disease as test positive. In other words, it is the probability of getting a positive test result when the disease is present. A highly sensitive test is rarely negative if disease is present, i.e., a highly sensitive test rarely misses individuals with the disease.

Specificity is the ability of a test to correctly classify individuals without the disease as test negative. In other words, it is the probability of getting a negative test result if the disease is absent. A highly specific test is rarely positive if the disease is absent.

The negative test result of a highly sensitive test is more important as it reduces the chance of a false negative, while the positive test result of a highly specific test is more important as it reduces the chance of a false positive. The confirmatory tests are highly specific.

The sensitivity and specificity of a test must be considered together because neither of them is very meaningful if considered singly. A highly sensitive test usually has low specificity (because of trade-offs between sensitivity and specificity; see Section 11.1.6). For example, a positive sputum culture for acid-fast bacilli (AFB) is a very specific test for the diagnosis of pulmonary tuberculosis, but it has low sensitivity.

11.1.3 Predictive Values

The sensitivity and specificity of a test help in selecting a test for screening or diagnosing a disease. Once a test is selected and applied to an individual (for the purpose of screening or diagnosis), it is important to know the positive and negative predictive values of the test. Positive and negative predictive values provide information about the usefulness of the test in practice.

The positive predictive value indicates the probability of having the disease in an individual when the test is positive, while the negative predictive value indicates the probability of not having the disease in an individual when the test is negative.

To calculate the sensitivity, specificity, and positive and negative predictive values, the test results (positive and negative) and disease status (present or absent) can be organized in a two-by-two table (Table 11.1). In this table, cell "a" represents the disease is present and the test is also positive (true positive; TP), while cell "d" represents the disease is absent and the test is negative (true negative; TN). Similarly, the cells "b (disease is absent but test is positive)" and "c (disease is present but test is negative)" indicate false positive (FP) and false negative (FN) test results, respectively.

The formulas (using the symbols from Table 11.1) to calculate the sensitivity, specificity, and positive and negative predictive values of a test are provided below:

$$\text{Sensitivity} = \frac{a}{(a+c)} \times 100$$

$$\text{Specificity} = \frac{d}{(b+d)} \times 100$$

$$\text{Positive predictive value} \ (+PV) = \frac{a}{(a+b)} \times 100$$

TABLE 11.1

Distribution of test results against a disease

	Disease		Total
	Present	**Absent**	**Total**
Test +ve	a (TP)	b (FP)	(a + b)
Test −ve	c (FN)	d (TN)	(c + d)
Total	(a + c)	(b + d)	(n)

Notes:　TP: True positive; FP: False positive; FN: False negative; TN: True negative

$$\text{Negative predictive value } (-PV) = \frac{d}{(c+d)} \times 100$$

The predictive values of a test can also be calculated if the sensitivity and specificity of the test and the prevalence of disease in the study population are known by using Bayes' theorem as follows:

$$\text{+ve Predictive Value} = \frac{P \times \text{Sensitivity}}{(P \times \text{Sensitivity}) + (1-P)(1-\text{Specificity})} \times 100$$

$$\text{−ve Predictive Value} = \frac{(1-P) \times \text{Specificity}}{(1-P)(\text{Specificity}) + P(1-\text{Sensitivity})} \times 100$$

Where P represents the prevalence of disease in the study population.

11.1.4 Efficiency

There is another term called the efficiency of a test. It is the summary statistic of the measure of validity of a test, considering both sensitivity and specificity together. Efficiency is the percentage of all true positive and true negative results of a test. It is calculated as:

$$\text{Efficiency} = \frac{(a+d)}{(a+b+c+d)} \times 100$$

If both sensitivity and specificity are high (i.e., the efficiency is high), the measure has high validity. Efficiency is sometimes used to compare the performance of two or more tests. The greater the measure of efficiency, the better the performance of the test.

There is another summary statistic called *Youden's J Statistic*. It is also a summary index of combined sensitivity and specificity, indicating the validity of a test. The J statistic is calculated as:

$$J = (\text{Sensitivity} + \text{Specificity}) - 1$$

For example, if the sensitivity and specificity of a test are 0.85 and 0.95, respectively, the value of J will be 0.80 (0.85 + 0.95 − 1) or 80%. Theoretically, the value of J ranges from -1 to +1. The value of J will be -1 if the sensitivity and specificity of the test are both zero. On the other hand, J will be equal to +1 if both the sensitivity and specificity of the test are 100%. However, a realistic minimum value of J is usually zero, which occurs when both sensitivity and specificity are 50%, meaning that the performance of the test is the worst.

The J statistic gives equal weight to sensitivity and specificity, indicating that both sensitivity and specificity are equally important for the measurement of the validity of a test.

11.1.5 Likelihood Ratios

Likelihood ratios (LRs) are measures that can be used to assess the overall performance of a test. It is another summary index that considers the sensitivity and specificity of the test together.

The LR can be calculated for both positive (LR +ve) and negative (LR −ve) tests. The LR for a positive test is the ratio of the probability of obtaining a positive test result when disease is present to the probability of a positive test result when disease is absent. Similarly, the LR for a negative test is the ratio of the probability of a negative test result when disease is present to the probability of a negative test result when disease is absent. The LR indicates how many times more (or less) likely it is to get a test result (positive or negative) in the presence of disease than in its absence. Likelihood ratios can be used to calculate the predictive values of a test. Likelihood ratios can be calculated by using the following formulas. Further details and uses of LRs can be seen elsewhere [4, 5].

LR for a positive test:

$$LR + ve = \frac{\text{Probability of a positive test result when disease is present}}{\text{Probability of a positive test result when disease is absent}}$$

Or (using the symbols of Table 11.1),

$$LR + ve = \frac{a \div (a + c)}{b \div (b + d)} \text{ or } \frac{\text{Sensitivity}}{(1 - \text{Specificity})}$$

On the other hand, LR for a negative test:

$$LR - ve = \frac{\text{Probability of a negative test result when disease is present}}{\text{Probability of a negative test result when disease is absent}}$$

Or,

$$LR - ve = \frac{c \div (a + c)}{d \div (b + d)} \text{ or } \frac{(1 - \text{Sensitivity})}{\text{Specificity}}$$

Example
Suppose that for a screening program, you want to evaluate the validity of the presence of blood in the stool for the screening of Shigellosis (bacillary

TABLE 11.2

Test results (presence of blood in stool) by Shigellosis

	Shigellosis		
	Present	Absent	Total
Test +ve (blood present)	195 (a)	60 (b)	255 (a + b)
Test –ve (blood absent)	105 (c)	240 (d)	345 (c + d)
Total	300 (a + c)	300 (b + d)	600 (n)

dysentery). To study the validity of the test (presence of blood in the stool), 300 individuals with Shigellosis (culture positive) and another 300 individuals without Shigellosis (culture negative) were selected. Among 300 individuals with Shigellosis, blood was present in the stools of 195 individuals, while blood was absent in the stools of 240 individuals who did not have Shigellosis. Data from the study are presented in Table 11.2. In this example, the screening test is "presence of blood in stool", and the test is being evaluated for the screening of patients with Shigellosis.

Using the formulas given earlier, we can calculate the:

$$\text{Sensitivity} = (195 \div 300) \times 100 = 65.0\%$$

$$\text{Specificity} = (240 \div 300) \times 100 = 80.0\%$$

$$\text{Positive predictive value} \left(+PV\right) = (195 \div 255) \times 100 = 76.5\%$$

$$\text{Negative predictive value} \left(-PV\right) = (240 \div 345) \times 100 = 69.5\%$$

$$\text{Efficiency} = \left[(195 + 240) \div 600\right] \times 100 = 72.5\%$$

$$\text{Youden's J} = (0.65 + 0.80) - 1 = 0.45$$

$$\text{LR +ve} = 0.65 \div (1 - 0.80) = 3.25$$

$$\text{LR -ve} = (1 - 0.65) \div 0.80 = 0.44$$

In our example, the sensitivity and specificity of the test are 65.0% and 80.0%, respectively. A sensitivity of 65.0% indicates that if disease (Shigellosis) is present, the probability of having blood in the stool is 65.0%. In other words, the chance of not having blood in the stool even if the person has Shigellosis is 35.0%. On the contrary, a specificity of 80.0% indicates that if the disease (Shigellosis) is absent, the probability of a negative test result (no blood in the stool) is 80.0%. This also indicates that 20% of patients without Shigellosis may have blood in the stool.

Sensitivity and specificity are proportions, and their confidence intervals (CIs) can be calculated from the data. For instance, the 95% CI of sensitivity can be calculated using the following formula:

$$95\% \text{ CI of sensitivity} = \text{Sensitivity} \pm \left(1.96 \times \text{Standard error (SE) of sensitivity}\right)$$

While the standard error (SE) of sensitivity is given by:

$$\text{SE of sensitivity} = \sqrt{\left(\frac{\text{Sensitivity} \times \left(1 - \text{Sensitivity}\right)}{\text{n}\left(\text{sample size}\right)}\right)}$$

From the data in Table 11.2, the SE of sensitivity is:

$$\text{SE of sensitivity} = \sqrt{\left(\frac{0.65 \times \left(1 - 0.65\right)}{300}\right)} = 0.028$$

Therefore, the 95% CI of sensitivity is:

$$95\% \text{ CI of sensitivity} = 0.65 \pm \left(1.96 \times 0.028\right); \text{i.e., } 0.60 - 0.71$$

The confidence interval indicates the range where the true sensitivity is likely to fall, with a certain level of confidence. In our example, the 95% CI for sensitivity is 0.60–0.71, indicating we are 95% confident that the actual sensitivity of the test in the population is likely to be between 0.60 and 0.71.

Similarly, to calculate the 95% CI for specificity from the data, use the same formulas, replacing the value for sensitivity with specificity. In our example, the 95% CI for specificity is 0.76–0.85.

Once the test is applied, it is important to know the positive and negative predictive values to understand the probabilities of having or not having the disease in an individual. A positive predictive value of 76.5% indicates that if the test is positive (i.e., blood is present in the stool), the probability of having Shigellosis is 76.5%. On the other hand, a negative predictive value of 69.5% indicates that when the test is negative (i.e., blood is absent in the stool) in an individual, the probability of not having Shigellosis is 69.5%.

The statistics for efficiency and Youden's J are summary statistics that are used to compare the performance of two or more tests. An LR +ve of 3.25 indicates that a positive test result is 3.25 times more likely to occur when the disease is present than when it is absent, while an LR −ve of 0.44 indicates the likelihood of obtaining a negative test result in the presence of the disease is 0.44 times that when it is absent.

11.1.6 Trade-Offs Between Sensitivity and Specificity

It is always desirable to find a test that is highly sensitive and highly specific for the screening program. In reality, such a test is not always possible to find. In general, there is always a trade-off between the sensitivity and specificity of a test. A trade-off is observed when the diagnosis is based on the test result of a continuous measurement, such as the blood sugar level for the diagnosis of diabetes mellitus or the serum glutamic-oxaloacetic transaminase (SGOT, also known as AST or aspartate aminotransferase) level for the diagnosis of acute myocardial infarction (MI). In such a situation, a cut-off value is used to separate out individuals who have the disease from those who do not.

For each cut-off point, the sensitivity and specificity of the test can be calculated. Depending on the cut-off point, one characteristic (e.g., sensitivity) can be increased (or decreased) at the expense of the other characteristic (specificity). Table 11.3 shows the trade-offs between sensitivity and specificity at different cut-off points of SGOT levels for the diagnosis of acute myocardial infarction (MI). The data (hypothetical) show that as the sensitivity decreases with the increase in cut-off value, there is an improvement in specificity.

11.1.7 ROC Curve

The trade-off between sensitivity and specificity of a test can be expressed by constructing the receiver operating characteristic (ROC) curve. The ROC curve is used to describe the accuracy of a test over a range of cut-off values. To construct the ROC curve, data on sensitivity is plotted against (100 − specificity) at different cut-off points. The ROC curve constructed using the data in Table 11.3 is illustrated in Figure 11.1.

TABLE 11.3

Sensitivity and specificity of serum glutamic-oxaloacetic transaminase (SGOT) levels (U/L), measured within six hours at different cut-off points for the diagnosis of acute myocardial infarction (hypothetical data)

Cut-off points (U/L)	Sensitivity (%)	Specificity (%)
44	100.0	0.0
50	100.0	4.0
60	100.0	14.0
70	100.0	30.0
80	98.0	58.0
90	88.0	84.0
100	74.0	94.0
110	52.0	98.0
120	26.0	100.0
130	14.0	100.0
140	8.0	100.0
146	0.0	100.0

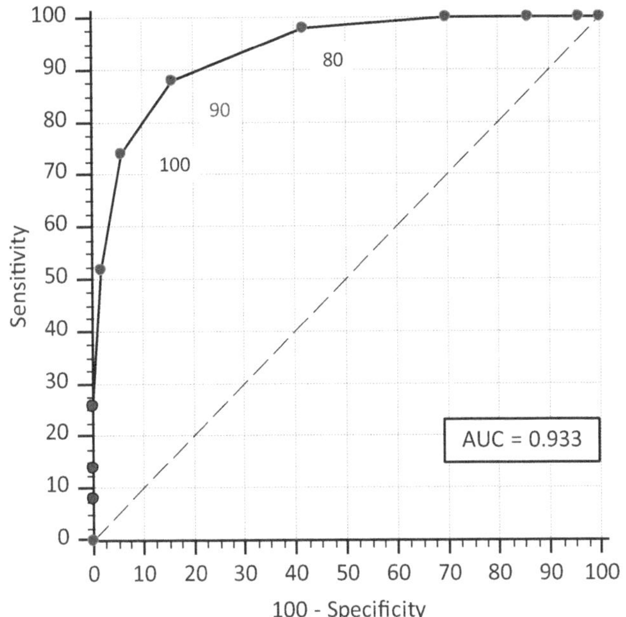

FIGURE 11.1

ROC curve to show the trade-off between sensitivity and specificity at different cut-off points of SGOT for the diagnosis of acute myocardial infarction. [Data from Table 11.3.]

The area under the ROC curve (AUC) is an important measure of a test's diagnostic performance. The area under the curve (AUC) ranges from zero to one. It indicates how good (or bad) the performance of a test is to distinguish between disease and non-disease. An AUC of 1.0 suggests perfect discrimination. In contrast, for a poorly performing test, the ROC curve lies closer to the diagonal line running from the lower left to the upper right corner. When AUC is 0.50, the ROC curve coincides with this diagonal line, suggesting that the performance of the test is no better than random chance in classifying disease status. The AUC can be used to compare the performance of two or more tests – the greater the AUC, the better the test's performance. In this example, the AUC is 0.933 (Figure 11.1), suggesting a strong ability of the test to differentiate MI from non-MI. The advantages of constructing the ROC curve are:

- It shows how severe the trade-off between sensitivity and specificity is for a test;
- Describes the accuracy (sensitivity and specificity) of a test over a range of cut-off points;
- Can be used to identify the best cut-off point for a test at which both sensitivity and specificity are high. The best cut-off point is the point that is

closest to the upper left corner. In our example, the best cut-off point is 90 U/L, where the sensitivity is 88.0% and the specificity is 84.0%;

- Serves as a nomogram for calculating the specificity that corresponds to a given sensitivity;
- To compare the accuracy of two or more tests (the greater the area under the curve, the better the test's ability to distinguish between disease and non-disease); and
- To calculate the likelihood ratios of a test at different cut-off points.

11.1.8 Relationship Between Prevalence and Predictive Values

Sensitivity and specificity are the inherent characteristics of a test. However, these characteristics may be affected by the way diseased (i.e., the spectrum of disease, such as severity and duration) and non-diseased individuals are selected for the evaluation of a test. Evaluation of a test is commonly done on individuals who clearly have the disease and on those who clearly do not have the disease. This means that only the extreme cases are involved in evaluating a test without considering the borderline cases (i.e., individuals who are in between normal and extreme cases). A test may have a greater ability to distinguish those who are clearly diseased from those who are not clearly diseased. Moreover, individuals with the disease in question may differ in severity, stage, or duration, and the sensitivity and specificity of a test may be higher in more severely affected individuals. As a result, the sensitivity and specificity of a test may be different in reality when it is applied to the general population for diagnosis or screening.

The predictive values of a test depend on its sensitivity and specificity, as well as the prevalence of the disease in the screened population. The positive predictive value increases as the disease prevalence increases, while the negative predictive value increases as the disease prevalence decreases.

The effects of prevalence on the positive and negative predictive values of a test with 90% sensitivity and 90% specificity are illustrated in Figure 11.2. At fixed sensitivity and specificity, if a test is applied to a population with a low prevalence of a disease, the positive predictive value will be lower than when it is applied to a population with a higher prevalence. Similarly, the negative predictive value will be higher in a situation where the prevalence of the disease is low. The figure illustrates that at 10% prevalence of a disease, the positive predictive value is only 50% for a test with 90% sensitivity and 90% specificity.

Example

In Soweto (South Africa), the prevalence of HIV among female sex workers (FSWs) is 53.6% [10], while it is less than 1% in Bangladesh. If we apply a screening test whose sensitivity and specificity are both 90%, the positive and negative predictive values of the test in Soweto and Bangladesh are shown in Table 11.4 (calculated by Bayes' theorem as described in Section 11.1.3). The

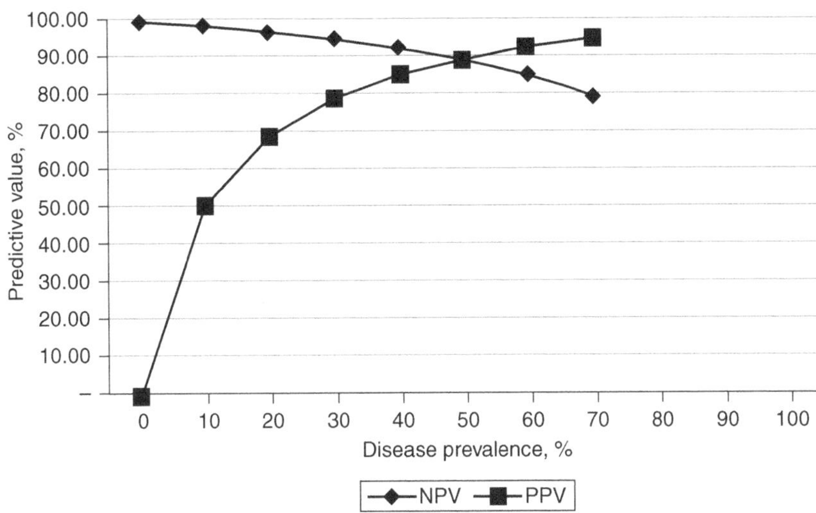

FIGURE 11.2

Positive and negative predictive values of a test with 90% sensitivity and 90% specificity according to the prevalence of disease.

Notes: PPV: Positive predictive value; NPV: Negative predictive value

TABLE 11.4

Positive and negative predictive values of an HIV screening test with 90% sensitivity and 90% specificity, applied to female sex workers in Soweto (HIV prevalence: 53.6%) and in Bangladesh (HIV prevalence: 1%)

Predictive value	Soweto	Bangladesh
+ve predictive value	91.2%	8.3%
-ve predictive value	88.6%	97.9%

results show that the positive predictive value of the test is more than 90.0% when it is applied to FSWs in Soweto (because of the high prevalence of HIV), compared to only about 8% when it is applied to FSWs in Bangladesh (because of the very low prevalence of HIV).

11.2 Screening in Health

11.2.1 Concept of Screening

The active search for a disease in apparently healthy individuals is a fundamental aspect of prevention. Screening is the search for an unrecognized disease (or a risk factor) by means of a rapidly applied test(s) (or an examination or other procedure) in *apparently healthy individuals.*

A screening test is not intended to be a diagnostic test. It is only an initial examination. Those who are found to be positive for a screening test are referred for confirmation of the disease with other test(s) and treatment. Screening is a preventive action, primarily a secondary prevention. Sometimes a screening test may be a diagnostic test, e.g., for hypertension and anemia.

The main purpose of screening is to sort out individuals from a group of apparently healthy people who are likely to have the disease and bring them under medical supervision and treatment. Screening is carried out with the assumption that early diagnosis and subsequent treatment will provide a better outcome.

11.2.2 Benefits and Risks of Screening

Screening has a number of benefits that include: a) early detection of disease can lead to improved outcomes; b) screening for an appropriate disease reduces mortality and morbidity; and c) screening is associated with increased quality of life and reduced costs of care. However, there are also risks associated with screening, such as: a) false-positive test results can lead to unnecessary anxiety, invasive follow-up testing, and treatment; b) false-negative test results can lead to delayed diagnosis and treatment; and c) harmful side effects of screening tests.

11.2.3 Objectives of Screening

Screening is primarily done for the early detection of disease, which may offer a better outcome. This objective is related to the direct benefit of individuals screened. For example, screening for cervical cancer and breast cancer among women. Screening is sometimes done for other purposes than the direct benefit of individuals being screened. They include [5]:

> *Compulsory screening of potential immigrants:* Screening for infectious diseases, such as tuberculosis, HIV, Hepatitis B, and other diseases, is done on prospective immigrants and migrant workers. Here, the objective of screening is to prevent the introduction of infectious diseases into a country to protect its own population. Obviously, this objective has low priority for the health benefits of individuals screened. Another example is the periodic health checkups of pilots to save airline passengers.

> *Screening for life insurance:* Screening is commonly done for some diseases when an individual wants to buy life insurance. In such a case, the company usually insists that the individual undergo physical examinations and some laboratory tests, especially to identify the

predictors (risk factors) of death, such as heart disease, diabetes, hypertension, or cancer. In this case, screening is primarily done for the financial protection of the insurance company rather than to improve the health of individuals.

Sometimes, screening is done to establish baseline data when the person is free from the disease.

11.2.4 Strategies for Screening

Early diagnosis through screening can be done in different ways. The commonly used strategies for screening are discussed below.

First, specified members of the *general public or a community* can be invited to undergo a specific test for the early diagnosis of a disease. For example, inviting the general public for blood pressure measurement to screen for hypertension, conducting a urine test to detect sugar for diabetes screening, or performing a visual inspection with acetic acid (VIA) for cervical cancer screening. Individuals found to be positive for the screening test are referred for confirmation of the disease and treatment. When multiple screening tests (e.g., blood pressure measurement and a urine test for sugar) are done in a single setting, it is called *multiphasic screening*. Such a strategy of screening at the community level is expensive and usually has low coverage.

The second strategy for screening is the *compulsory and periodic medical checkup*. For example, compulsory screening is commonly done for pilots, while periodic medical checkups can be done for staff of an organization (e.g., all icddr,b staff undergo a medical checkup once every three years). This type of screening targets a specific group of people rather than the general population.

Third, screening can be done on individuals when they visit their physicians for a specific condition. The physician can take the opportunity to screen patients for other conditions, such as measurement of blood pressure for hypertension and blood sugar testing for diabetes. Such a strategy, where doctors take the opportunity to screen individuals for other conditions than the specific problem during the visit, is called *case finding*. For example, a physician may screen a patient for diabetes, hypertension, or breast cancer when the patient presents with a respiratory tract infection. Such a strategy is less expensive and is suitable where the majority of people visit their physician once or twice a year (e.g., 75% of Canadians visit a physician once a year).

11.2.5 Selecting a Test for Screening

It is always important to select a suitable test for screening. The screening test(s) to be selected for a screening program should have reasonably high sensitivity and specificity. The other criteria for selecting a test are low cost, ease of administration, safety, imposing minimal discomfort upon administration, and acceptability to the community and providers. Though it is desirable to use a test that is highly sensitive and highly specific, it may not be possible to find such a test in reality. A screening test usually has high sensitivity but low specificity, or high specificity but low sensitivity. In a situation where a choice has to be made between a sensitive and a specific test, the decision depends on the purpose of the screening program. A highly *sensitive test* is recommended when:

- The disease is serious, should not be missed, and effective treatment is available;
- The disease may create a public health problem through its rapid spread;
- Subsequent diagnostic tests can be done with minimal cost and risk; and
- A false positive test result does not cause social and psychological trauma to individuals.

On the other hand, a highly *specific test* is more realistic when:

- The disease is some sort of social stigma;
- The confirmatory test is complicated, expensive, physically traumatic, or risky; and
- There is an effective treatment for the disease.

11.2.6 Use of Multiple Tests in Screening

Commonly, a highly sensitive and highly specific test is difficult to find for a screening program. In such cases, a combination of tests can be used to enhance either the overall sensitivity or specificity of the available tests, as individual tests alone do not provide satisfactory efficiency. There are two methods of using multiple tests in combination.

a) *Combination in series:* In this method, if the first test is positive, the second (and subsequent) test is used. The result of a combination in series is considered positive when both test results are positive (Table 11.5). A positive test result in a series increases the specificity when considered together.

b) *Combination in parallel:* In this method, both tests are administered simultaneously. If any of the test results are positive, the overall test is considered positive. The result is considered negative when both test results are negative (Table 11.5). A positive test result in parallel increases the sensitivity in combination.

The overall sensitivity and specificity of a combination of tests (e.g., test A and test B) can be calculated using the following formulas:

TABLE 11.5

Interpretation of tests in combination

Individual test results		Conclusion in combination	
Test A	Test B	Test in series	Test in parallel
Positive	Positive	Positive	Positive
Positive	Negative	Negative	Positive
Negative	Positive	Negative	Positive
Negative	Negative	Negative	Negative

Test in series

$$\text{Overall sensitivity} = (\text{Sensitivity of test A}) \times (\text{Sensitivity of test B})$$

$$\text{Overall specificity} = 1 - \left[(1 - \text{Specificity of test A}) \times (1 - \text{Specificity of test B})\right]$$

Test in parallel

$$\text{Overall sensitivity} = 1 - \left[(1 - \text{Sensitivity of test A}) \times (1 - \text{Sensitivity of test B})\right]$$

$$\text{Overall specificity} = (\text{Specificity of test A}) \times (\text{Specificity of test B})$$

Example

Suppose an investigator has selected two tests (Test A and Test B) for a screening program. The sensitivity and specificity of Test A are 75% and 80%, respectively, while those of Test B are 80% and 70%, respectively. What will be the overall sensitivity and specificity of these tests when they are applied together in series and in parallel?

The overall sensitivity and specificity of the tests when applied together in series:

$$\text{Overall sensitivity} = (0.75) \times (0.80) = 0.60 \text{ or } 60.0\%$$

$$\text{Overall specificity} = 1 - \left[(1 - 0.80) \times (1 - 0.70)\right] = 0.94 \text{ or } 94.0\%$$

The overall sensitivity and specificity of the tests when applied together in parallel:

$$\text{Overall sensitivity} = 1 - \left[(1 - 0.75) \times (1 - 0.80)\right] = 0.95 \text{ or } 95.0\%$$

$$\text{Overall specificity} = (0.80) \times (0.70) = 0.56 \text{ or } 56\%$$

11.2.7 Diseases Suitable for Screening

A screening program is said to be effective if the detection of a disease in its pre-symptomatic stage reduces morbidity and mortality from the disease. Diseases and risk factors that are commonly screened for early diagnosis include breast cancer and cervical cancer in women, colorectal cancer, diabetes, high blood pressure, high cholesterol, osteoporosis, overweight and obesity, and prostate cancer in men.

To understand which disease is suitable for screening, it is essential to clearly understand the natural history of the disease. The natural history of a disease refers to the progression of the disease process in an individual over time in the absence of intervention. Events that occur in the natural history of a disease over time are divided into four stages (Figure 11.3) [4, 5, 11].

> *Biological onset:* The process of the occurrence of a disease begins with exposure to or accumulation of factors sufficient to initiate a disease in a susceptible host. This is the initial stage of the disease. At this stage, there are no clinical manifestations (symptoms or signs), and the disease cannot be detected by a screening or diagnostic test. At this stage, the disease remains undetected.
>
> *Preclinical stage:* With the passage of time after the biological onset, the disease causes some structural and functional changes in the host, though the individual remains free from symptoms. At this stage, early diagnosis is possible if an appropriate test is applied through screening programs, case findings, or periodic health examinations. The time interval between this stage and the point of "clinical stage", when the disease can be detected by a screening or diagnostic test, is sometimes referred to as the *detectable preclinical phase.*
>
> *Clinical stage:* As the disease progresses, the person develops clinical manifestations (signs and symptoms) at a particular point and becomes

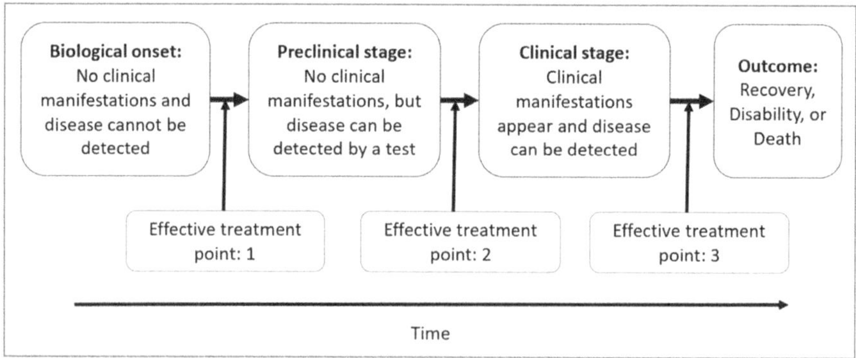

FIGURE 11.3

Stages of the natural history of the disease process and effective treatment points in it.

ill. This is the clinical stage of the disease, when patients usually come to doctors and seek medical care. Diagnosis of a disease is commonly made at this stage. This stage is sometimes called the stage of "usual clinical diagnosis".

Outcome: Finally, the disease progresses on its own course, either spontaneously or due to interventions. The outcome of a disease may be spontaneous recovery (e.g., the majority of hepatitis A infections recover spontaneously), disability (e.g., most polio cases have spontaneous recovery, but a few may end up with paralysis), or death.

It is assumed that there are some critical points in the course of the natural history of disease (Figure 11.3). The critical points are the points before which treatment is more effective. A disease may have several critical points spread over its natural history, or it may have none. If the disease's critical point is in between biological onset and the preclinical stage (i.e., at effective treatment point 1, as shown in Figure 11.3) when the disease cannot be detected, it is already too late to help the patient through a screening program. Since the point of effective treatment is before the stage of early diagnosis through screening, the opportunity for effective treatment is lost.

If the critical point is at "effective treatment point 3", it may be too early to detect the disease by screening using manpower, money, and other resources. Since the effective treatment point is between the clinical stage and outcome, it may be prudent to wait until the patient develops clinical manifestations for diagnosis and treatment.

Therefore, screening for a disease is only effective if the critical point lies between the "preclinical stage " and "clinical stage" of the natural history of the disease, i.e., at "effective treatment point 2". The criteria for diseases suitable for a screening program include [12]:

- Diseases for which there is evidence that treatment in the preclinical (early) stage is more effective than treatment begun after the development of symptoms. For example, the screening for cervical cancer in women;

- Diseases that are often fatal, such as breast cancer, and those known to have serious and irreversible consequences (e.g., congenital hypothyroidism) if not treated early;

- The disease should be fairly prevalent in the screened population. This relates to the positive predictive value (Section 11.1.3) and cost of the screening program in terms of the number of cases detected;

- In some cases, screening for a disease with a low prevalence may be cost-effective when the cost of the screening program is less than the cost of care if the disease is not detected early. For example, phenylketonuria (PKU) is a rare disease (the estimated prevalence is about one in 15,000 births) but has very serious long-term consequences if left untreated. In a situation like this, screening may be justified;

- A suitable screening test is available. Suitability criteria refer to adequate sensitivity and specificity, low cost, ease of administration, safety, imposing minimal discomfort upon administration, and being acceptable to providers and pfigicipants; and

- There must be an appropriate follow-up for individuals who are positive for the screening test for confirmation of the diagnosis.

For example, the disease hypertension fulfills all the criteria for screening. First, hypertension is a serious disease associated with higher morbidity and premature death. Second, early detection and effective treatment reduce morbidity and mortality due to hypertension. Third, the prevalence of hypertension is reasonably high (overall prevalence is 21% among the age group 18–69 years in Bangladesh) [13] in the target population for screening.

11.2.8 Criteria for Screening Programs

The World Health Organization (WHO) published guidelines on the principles and practice of screening for diseases, which are often referred to as the Wilson and Jungner criteria [14]. The major criteria for a screening program, as outlined by the WHO, include:

- The condition (disease) should be an important public health problem;
- There should be a treatment for the condition;
- Facilities for diagnosis and treatment should be available;
- There should be a latent stage of the disease;
- There should be a suitable screening test or examination for the condition;
- The screening test should be acceptable to the population;
- The natural history of the disease should be adequately understood;
- There should be an agreed policy on whom to treat;
- The total cost of finding a case should be economically balanced in relation to medical expenditure as a whole; and
- Case-finding should be a continuous process, not just a "once and for all" project.

11.2.9 Potential Sources of Bias in the Evaluation of a Screening Program

To evaluate a screening program, two groups of people are required: one group of people who are diagnosed based on screening (the screening group) and another group of people who are diagnosed based on the development of symptoms (the unscreened group). Both groups must be similar with regard to all factors affecting the outcome under evaluation except for screening experience. While evaluating a screening program, it is important to be aware of three sources of potential bias. They include volunteer bias, lead-time bias, and length-time bias [2–5].

11.2.9.1 Volunteer Bias or Selection Bias

When an observational study is designed to evaluate a screening program, the study subjects are selected from those who are willing to participate (volunteers) in the study. People who opt to participate (volunteers) in a screening program are likely to be different from those who do not volunteer in different ways that may affect the outcome under investigation. In general, volunteers are more health-conscious, have better health, and are more likely to adhere to interventions than the general population. As a result, if an observational study is designed, it is more likely that the screened group will have a better probability of survival (a lower mortality rate) than nonparticipants (the unscreened group), regardless of the effectiveness of the screening program.

Selection bias may be avoided by designing a randomized trial. In this design, the participants are randomized into screening and non-screening groups, and the prognosis after diagnosis is evaluated over time. Such a design is efficient in improving the internal validity but potentially limits the external validity (because of the selection of a specific group).

11.2.9.2 Lead-Time Bias

Lead-time bias occurs when there is a better prognosis (e.g., survival probability) for cases detected by the screening procedure than for cases diagnosed by the normal clinical procedure without adjusting for lead-time. Lead time is the interval between the diagnosis of a disease at the point of screening (using a screening test) and the diagnosis of the disease at the point of development of symptoms. Therefore, individuals who are in the screening group will have their diagnosis earlier by some amount of time compared to those who are in the unscreened group. The lead-time varies from disease to disease and from individual to individual. If this element of lead-time is not taken into consideration, the survival probability may be erroneously higher among individuals in the screened group than in the unscreened group.

There are two ways to control this bias. First, when the lead-time for the disease can be estimated (from other studies), it can be taken into consideration during analysis by deducting this time from subjects in the screening group. The second is to analyze the data to compare the age-specific mortality rates in screened and unscreened groups rather than the survival experiences between screened and unscreened (detected by clinical symptoms) groups.

11.2.9.3 Length-Time Bias

Diseases tend to be heterogeneous with respect to their natural history. It is evident that some cancers grow faster and others, even in the same organ, grow much more slowly. Patients with a long preclinical phase of a disease usually have a longer clinical phase and a better survival probability than patients with a shorter preclinical phase of the disease. Patients with a long preclinical phase are more likely to be detected by screening than those with a short preclinical phase. As a result, more cases with a short preclinical duration are left for the unscreened group (i.e., the group diagnosed at the time of the development of clinical manifestations). This leads to better survival for screened cases, even though screening is not beneficial. Such a phenomenon is called the length-time bias.

References

1.   Park JE, Park K. *Textbook of Preventive and Social Medicine*. 12th ed. Jabalpur: M/S Banarsidas Bhanot; 1989.
2.   Gordis L. *Epidemiology*. 5th ed. Philadelphia: Elsevier Saunders; 2014.
3.   Hennekens CH, Buring JE. *Epidemiology in Medicine*. Boston/Toronto: Little Brown and Company; 1987.
4.   Fletcher RH, Fletcher SW, Wagner EH. *Clinical Epidemiology: The Essentials*. 2nd ed. Philadelphia, US: Williams & Wilkins; 1988.
5.   Sackett DL, Haynes RB, Guyatt GH, Tugwell P. *Clinical Epidemiology: A Basic Science for Clinical Medicine*. 2nd ed. Boston/Toronto/London: Little, Brown and Company; 1991.
6.   Mausner JS, Kramer S. *Epidemiology: An Introductory Text*. 2nd ed. Philadelphia: WB Saunders Company; 1985.
7.   Supanvanich S, Podhipak A. *Principles of Epidemiology*. Thailand: Faculty of Public Health, Mahidol University; 1991.
8.   Persson LA, Wall S. *Epidemiology for Public Health*. Sweden: Umea University; 2000.
9.   Katz MH. *Study Design and Statistical Analysis: A Practical Guide for Clinicians*. Cambridge: Cambridge University Press; 2009.
10. Coetzee J, Jewkes R, Gray GE. Cross-sectional study of female sex workers in Soweto, South Africa: Factors associated with HIV infection. *PLoS ONE*. 2017;12(10):e0184775. doi:10.1371/journal.pone.0184775
11. Centers for Disease Control and Prevention (CDC). *Lesson 1: Introduction to Epidemiology, Section 9: Natural History and Spectrum of Disease*; 2023. Available from: https://archive.cdc.gov/www_cdc_gov/csels/dsepd/ss1978/lesson1/section9.html
12. New York State Department of Health. *Screening for Chronic Diseases*; 1999. Available from www.health.ny.gov/diseases/chronic/discreen.htm#:~:text=What%20criteria%20should%20be%20considered,hypothyroidism%2C%20are%20appropriate%20for%20screening

13. National Institute of Preventive and Social Medicine (NIPSOM). *National STEPS Survey for Non-communicable Diseases Risk Factors in Bangladesh.* Bangladesh: Ministry of Health and Family Welfare; 2018.

14. Wilson JMG, Jungner G. Principles and practice of screening for disease. *WHO Chronicle.* 1968; 22(11):281–393.

12

Measures of Agreement

Mohammad Tajul Islam

Health workers spend a significant portion of their time measuring various individual characteristics. These measurements are closely linked to decision-making in patient management or drawing conclusions from research. Overall, the characteristics measured can be broadly classified as exposure (or predictor) factors and outcome (or effect) factors.

In health research, investigators have to rely on multiple people for data collection from study subjects. The issue of consistency among individuals collecting data arises due to the inherent variability among human observers. Variables subjected to interobserver (interrater) variations are commonly found in clinical (e.g., clinical diagnosis of a patient or findings from an X-ray plate) and laboratory (e.g., platelet counts) studies. A well-designed research study must address the variability of measurements among data collectors to ensure data quality and draw valid conclusions.

Common sources of variation in measurements include a) observer variation, such as interobserver (between observers) and intraobserver (within an observer) variation; b) variation due to instruments, such as the same instrument may give different readings when repeated, and there may be differences in readings between instruments; and c) biological variability within subjects (also see Section 11.1.1).

Variability in measurements is usually minimized through the training of data collectors and checking how consistently they record the observations. In reality, perfect consistency (agreement) among data collectors is rare, and the validity of study results depends partly on the level of consistency among data collectors. The extent to which data collectors agree on the measurement of an outcome or exposure variable can be categorized as: a) interrater (interobserver) reliability, indicating reliability (agreement) across multiple data collectors on the same subjects under the same conditions; and b) intrarater (intraobserver) reliability, indicating reliability of a single data collector on the same subject on different occasions.

DOI: 10.1201/9781003654803-12

If a variable has only two clearly defined outcomes, agreement is likely to be high. For example, in a study of survival after an acute heart attack, the outcome is either "survived" or "died". However, when data collectors must make finer distinctions, such as severity of anemia (e.g., no, mild, moderate, or severe anemia) in pregnant women, achieving agreement is much more difficult. Measuring the extent of agreement on the variables of interest is essential to ensuring data quality and drawing a valid conclusion.

12.1 Measurement of Interrater Reliability

Agreement (reliability) between two observers (raters) or measurements can be assessed for either a categorical variable or a continuous variable. The choice of statistical method for the assessment depends on the type of variable (whether categorical or continuous) being evaluated and the number of observers (raters) involved in the measurements. Table 12.1 summarizes the methods of agreement analysis depending on the type of variable and the number of raters involved in the measurements [1].

Besides the statistical methods shown in Table 12.1, there are several other methods that are used to measure the interrater (interobserver) and intrarater (intraobserver) reliability. Some of these methods include percent agreement, Pearson's correlation coefficient (r), and Krippendorff's alpha (useful when there are multiple raters and multiple possible ratings) [1–3]. The focus in the measurement of interrater reliability is on the extent to which two (or more) raters agree, rather than their relationship with a gold standard or true outcome [2, 4, 5].

TABLE 12.1

Methods used for the assessment of agreement between observers or methods

Type of variable	No. of raters or methods	Method for agreement analysis
Categorical (nominal)	Two	Cohen's kappa
	More than two	Fleiss' kappa
Categorical (ordinal)	Two	Weighted kappa
	More than two	Fleiss' kappa
Continuous	Two or more	Bland-Altman plot with limits of agreement; Intra-class correlation coefficient (ICC).

12.2 Agreement Between Two Raters on a Categorical Outcome

12.2.1 Percent Agreement

Suppose a researcher is interested in estimating BCG vaccine (for tuberculosis) coverage among children under five years of age in a community. It is decided to use the presence (or absence) of a BCG scar on the arms to assess children's BCG vaccination status. To collect data, the researcher employed two data collectors (raters). To evaluate the agreement (interrater reliability) in the ascertainment of BCG scars by two data collectors, the researcher selected 200 children, some of whom had BCG scars while others did not. These 200 children were independently examined by both data collectors and recorded their observations on the presence or absence of BCG scars. The results are presented in Table 12.2.

- Data in cell "a" indicates both raters (data collectors) agreed on the presence of BCG scars (concordant cell);
- Data in cell "b" indicates rater 1 said the BCG scar was absent, while rater 2 said the scar was present, i.e., two raters disagreed on the presence (or absence) of the BCG scar (discordant cell);
- Data in cell "C" indicates rater 1 said the BCG scar was present, while rater 2 said the scar was absent, i.e., two raters disagreed on the presence (or absence) of the BCG scar (discordant cell); and
- Data in cell "d" indicates both raters agreed on the absence of BCG scars (concordant cell).

From the table (Table 12.2), we can see that the two data collectors agreed on having a BCG scar in 140 children (cell "a") and did not have a BCG scar in 30 children (cell "d"). Therefore, the proportion (%) of agreement among two data collectors is:

$$\text{Percent agreement} = \frac{a+d}{n} \text{ or } \frac{140+30}{200} = 0.85 \text{ or } 85.0\%$$

TABLE 12.2

Observations of two data collectors on the presence of BCG scars in 200 children

		Data collector 1		Total
		Scar present	Scar absent	
Data collector 2	Scar present	140 (a)	10 (b)	**150 (R1)**
	Scar absent	20 (c)	30 (d)	**50 (R2)**
	Total	**160 (C1)**	**40 (C2)**	**200 (n)**

The percent agreement in this example indicates that in 85% of instances, both data collectors agree on the status of BCG vaccination. Conversely, it can be said that 85% of the data are reliable and 15% are invalid because, when there is no agreement, only one of the data collectors will be correct.

The percent agreement statistic is easy to calculate and interpret directly. However, its key limitation is that it does not account for the possibility that raters might agree to some extent by chance (since we expect some agreement between the raters even if they were guessing). As a result, it may over-estimate the true agreement between two raters. One way to address this problem is to use Cohen's kappa statistic [2, 4, 5].

12.2.2 Cohen's Kappa

Cohen's kappa, commonly referred to as kappa, is denoted by the Greek letter κ. Kappa statistic or kappa coefficient is widely used to assess the degree of agreement between two raters (observers) or methods on a categorical variable with two or more levels (categories) in health research [2, 5]. It can also be extended to more than two raters (Fleiss' kappa).

Kappa quantifies the extent to which two raters (or methods) agree on a categorical variable that they measure independently, taking into account the agreement occurring by chance, i.e., kappa is a measure of chance-corrected proportional agreement. Kappa is used when two raters independently assess whether a condition (e.g., a disease, a clinical manifestation, or others) is present or absent using the same criteria. Kappa is calculated using the data in the diagonal cells (concordant cells), which represent complete agreement between two raters. It does not take into account the discordant cells (cells where the two raters do not agree). The formula for the kappa statistic is:

$$\kappa = \frac{P_O - P_e}{1 - P_e}$$

Where P_0 represents the proportion of observed agreement and P_e is the proportion of expected agreement by chance.

The percent agreement (85%, or 0.85) that was calculated earlier is the proportion of observed agreement (P_0). Let us use the data from Table 12.2 to calculate the kappa coefficient (κ). To calculate the kappa coefficient, we need to calculate the proportion of expected agreement (P_e) between two raters by chance, which is calculated based on the expected values for cells "a" and "d". To calculate the expected values for cells "a" and "d", use the following formula (it is the same formula that we use to calculate the expected values for a chi-square test in a k-by-k table):

$$\text{Expected value for cell "a"} = \frac{C1 \times R1}{n} \text{ or } \frac{160 \times 150}{200} = 120$$

TABLE 12.3

Guideline for interpretation of kappa coefficient

Value of kappa	Strength of agreement
≤ 0	Poor agreement
$0.01 - 0.20$	Slight agreement
$0.21 - 0.40$	Fair agreement
$0.41 - 0.60$	Moderate agreement
$0.61 - 0.80$	Substantial agreement
$0.81 - 1.0$	Almost perfect agreement

$$\text{Expected value for cell "d"} = \frac{C2 \times R2}{n} \text{ or } \frac{40 \times 50}{200} = 10$$

$$\text{Proportion of expected agreement by chance} \left(p_e\right) = \frac{120 + 10}{200} = 0.65$$

Therefore,

$$\text{Kappa,} \; \kappa = \frac{0.85 - 0.65}{1 - 0.65} = 0.5714$$

Theoretically, the value of kappa ranges from -1 to +1, though commonly it falls between zero and +1. A kappa value of +1 indicates perfect agreement between two raters; zero indicates agreement no better than expected by chance; and a negative value indicates agreement worse than that expected by chance. Landis and Koch [3, 6] proposed guidelines for interpreting kappa statistics, as shown in Table 12.3. In general, a kappa value of less than 0.60 should be considered inadequate agreement among raters [4]. In our example, kappa is 0.57, indicating a moderate agreement between the data collectors.

12.2.3 Confidence Interval of Kappa

One can calculate the confidence interval (CI) for kappa. The formula for the calculation of the 95% CI of kappa is:

$$95\% \text{ CI of } \kappa = \kappa \pm 1.96 \times \text{Standard error of } \kappa$$

Here, 1.96 is the two-sided Z-value corresponding to a 95% confidence level. The standard error (SE) of kappa is given by:

$$\text{SE (standard error) of } \kappa = \sqrt{\frac{p_o\left(1 - p_o\right)}{n\left(1 - p_e\right)^2}}$$

Where P_0 is the proportion of observed agreement, P_e is the proportion of expected agreement by chance, and n is the sample size. In our example, the values for P_0, P_e, and n are 0.85, 0.65, and 200, respectively.
The SE of kappa for the data in Table 12.2 is:

$$\text{SE (standard error) of } \kappa = \sqrt{\frac{0.85(1-0.85)}{200(1-0.65)^2}} = 0.0721$$

Therefore, the 95% CI for kappa is 0.4328 – 0.7154, as shown below:

$$95\% \text{ CI of } \kappa = (0.5714 \pm 1.96 \times 0.0721) \text{ or } 0.4328 \text{ to } 0.7154$$

The confidence interval indicates the range where the true kappa value is likely to fall, with a certain level of confidence. In our example, the 95% CI for kappa is 0.43 – 0.72, meaning we are 95% confident that the actual agreement between two raters is likely to be between 0.43 and 0.72.

12.2.4 Weighted Kappa: Agreement Between Two Raters on an Ordinal Categorical Outcome

Kappa can also be calculated to evaluate the agreement between two raters (or methods) when the categorical outcome variable has more than two categories (such as data from three-by-three, four-by-four, or k-by-k tables), as shown in Table 12.4 [7, 8]. In our example (Table 12.4), the outcome variable is the presence and severity of a murmur (an abnormal heart sound commonly caused by damaged heart valves) in 160 patients, which is an

TABLE 12.4

Data from 160 patients with heart disease evaluated by two physicians (raters) for the presence and intensity of a murmur

Rater 2	Rater 1				
	No murmur	Mild murmur	Moderate murmur	Severe murmur	Total
No murmur	40 (a) [19.5]	10 (b)	2 (c)	0 (d)	52
Mild murmur	15 (e)	25 (f) [12.6]	7 (g)	1 (h)	48
Moderate murmur	5 (i)	5 (j)	15 (k) [7.0]	10 (l)	35
Severe murmur	0 (m)	2 (n)	8 (o)	15 (p) [4.1]	25
Total	60	42	32	26	160

Notes: Numbers in [] are the expected frequencies.

ordinal categorical variable with four levels (no, mild, moderate, and severe murmur), evaluated by two doctors (raters).

In this example, the unweighted proportions of observed and chance agreements are 0.59 and 0.27, respectively, as shown below.

$$\text{Unweighted proportion of observed agreement } \left(p_o\right)$$

$$= \frac{40+25+15+15}{160} = 0.59$$

$$\text{Unwighted proportion of chance agreement } \left(p_e\right)$$

$$= \frac{19.5+12.6+7.0+4.1}{160} = 0.27$$

Therefore,

$$\text{Unweighted } \kappa = \frac{0.59-0.27}{1-0.27} = 0.44$$

An unweighted kappa of 0.44 indicates moderate agreement between the two raters. A weakness of the unweighted kappa is that it does not account for the degree of disagreement, i.e., all disagreements are treated equally. Weighted kappa addresses this by assigning weights to the data in all cells.

When the categories of a variable are ordered (such as no murmur, mild murmur, moderate murmur, and severe murmur), it may be preferable to assign different weights to cells with disagreements, considering the magnitude of the discrepancy. The weights are assigned to each cell according to its distance from the diagonal cell (i.e., cells a, f, k, and p), which indicates complete agreement. Here, observations next to the diagonal cells (cells in which both raters agree) represent a difference of only one category and are less serious than those where the discrepancies are two or three categories apart. Note that weighted kappa is only used when the categorical outcome is an ordinal variable (it is not logical to use weighted kappa for a nominal variable).

For example, referring to the data in Table 12.4, the difference in raters' observations between "no murmur" and "mild murmur" is less serious than the difference between "no murmur" and "moderate or severe murmur". As a result, less weight (for agreement) is given to discrepancies that are further apart from the diagonal cells, indicating complete agreement (i.e., cells a, f, k, and p).

There are several different ways to weight the kappa statistic, depending on the specific situation and the type of data to be analyzed. Commonly used weighting schemes include linear and quadratic weight [9]. The formula for the calculation of linear weight for the kappa statistic is given by [7, 9]:

$$\text{Weight for } \kappa = 1 - \frac{|I - J|}{G - 1}$$

Where "I" represents the row number, "J" represents the corresponding column number for a cell, and "G" represents the number of categories in the outcome variable. For example, in Table 12.4, for cell "b", the value for "I" is one (row 1), the value for "J" is two (column 2), and the value for "G" is four (since there are four categories in the variable measured). Therefore, the weight for cell "b" is 0.67. In the same manner, we can assign weights to each cell to calculate the weighted kappa. Table 12.5 shows the weight assigned (denoted by "W") to each cell using the above formula. Note that the assignment of weights to cells is somewhat arbitrary. It should be decided on the basis of the investigator's perception of how serious the disagreement is in the context of the study objective.

Using the assigned weights, one can calculate the weighted kappa. Let us use the data from Table 12.5 to calculate the weighted kappa.

To calculate the weighted proportion of observed agreement (weighted P_0): a) first, multiply the observed frequencies in all cells by their corresponding weights; b) sum all the resulting products; and c) finally, divide the sum by the grand total. Similarly, to calculate the weighted proportion of chance agreement (weighted P_e): a) multiply the expected frequencies in all cells by their corresponding weights; b) sum all the resulting products; and c) divide the sum by the grand total. Finally, calculate the weighted kappa using the

TABLE 12.5

Weights assigned to each cell for the data presented in Table 12.4

Rater 2	Rater 1				
	No murmur	Mild murmur	Moderate murmur	Severe murmur	Total
No murmur	O=40 E=19.5 W=1	O=10 E=13.7 W=0.67	O=2 E=10.4 W=0.33	O=0 E=8.5 W=0	52
Mild murmur	O=15 E=18.0 W=0.67	O=25 E=12.6 W=1	O=7 E=7.0 W=0.67	O=1 E=7.8 W=0.33	48
Moderate murmur	O=5 E=13.1 W=0.33	O=5 E=9.2 W=0.67	O=15 E=7.0 W=1	O=10 E=5.7 W=0.67	35
Severe murmur	O=0 E=9.4 W=0	O=2 E=6.6 W=0.33	O=8 E=5.0 W=0.67	O=15 E=4.1 W=1	25
Total	60	42	32	26	160

Notes: O: Observed frequency; E: Expected frequency; and W: Weight.

formula for the kappa statistic as shown in Section 12.2.2. Readers interested in the formula for the weighted kappa are referred to [7].

Weighted proportion of observed agreement (weighted P_0):

$$[(40 + 25 + 15 + 15) \times 1 + (10 + 7 + 10 + 15 + 5 + 8) \times 0.67 + (2 + 1 + 5 + 2) \times 0.33 + (0 + 0) \times 0] \div 160 = 0.84$$

Weighted proportion of chance agreement (weighted P_e):

$$[(19.5 + 12.6 + 7.0 + 4.1) \times 1 + (13.7 + 7.0 + 5.7 + 18.0 + 9.2 + 5.0) \times 0.67 + (10.4 + 7.8 + 13.1 + 6.6) \times 0.33 + (9.4 + 8.5) \times 0] \div 160 = 0.59$$

$$\text{Weighted } \kappa = \frac{0.84 - 0.59}{1 - 0.59} = 0.62$$

The weighted kappa calculated from the data is 0.62, indicating substantial agreement between the two raters (Table 12.3). This value is higher than the unweighted kappa of 0.44 that we calculated earlier. In general, the weighted kappa provides a better estimate of agreement than the unweighted kappa, but it can only be used with data on an ordinal scale with at least three categories [3].

12.2.5 Limitations of Kappa

There are several limitations associated with the use and interpretation of kappa. The most common problem is that the value of kappa depends on the prevalence of the condition. In our example (Table 12.2), the proportion (prevalence) of children with the BCG vaccine (both agreed) is 70%. If the prevalence changes (either increases or decreases), the kappa value will also change. As a consequence of this property, it is misleading to compare kappa values from different studies where the prevalence differs. Another issue is that kappa also depends on the number of categories in the exposure or outcome variable. The kappa value is generally greater if there are fewer categories, and its value tends to be relatively high when there are only two categories [3, 7, 8].

12.3 Agreement Between Two Continuous Data (Quantitative Outcomes)

Agreement between two measurements (by two raters, methods, or instruments) on continuous data can be assessed statistically. Suppose two doctors measured the systolic blood pressure (BP) of 20 individuals using the same instrument and under the same conditions. The data are presented in Table 12.6 (hypothetical data). We will use this data to evaluate the agreement between the two raters (doctors) for the measurement of systolic BP.

12.3.1 Pearson's Correlation Coefficient

The simplest way to compare two sets of measurements on a continuous variable is to construct a scatter diagram. Figure 12.1 shows the scatter diagram of the data in Table 12.6. If raters (doctors) had complete agreement, the data points would lie on the line of equality (as shown in the figure), which is the 45° diagonal line from the origin. The figure shows that although the data

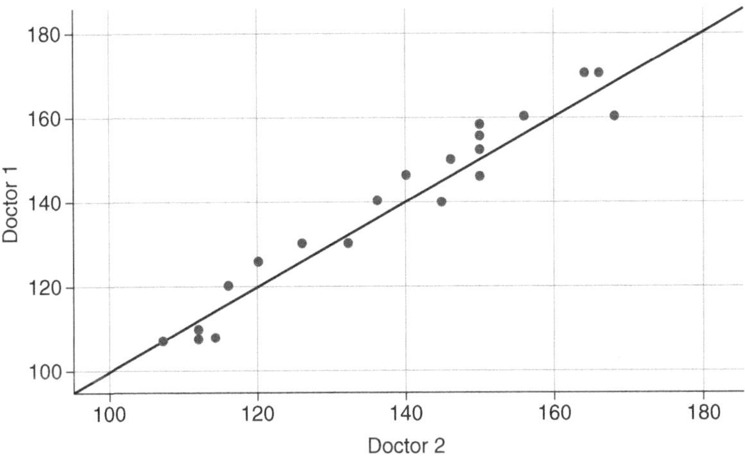

FIGURE 12.1

Scatter diagram of systolic bold pressure measured by two doctors.

TABLE 12.6

Systolic BP (mmHg) of 20 individuals measured by two doctors

Subject	Doctor 1	Doctor 2	Subject	Doctor 1	Doctor 2
1.	107	107	11.	150	146
2.	108	114	12.	155	150
3.	110	112	13.	146	150
4.	108	112	14.	158	150
5.	126	120	15.	160	156
6.	130	126	16.	160	168
7.	130	132	17.	140	136
8.	120	116	18.	170	166
9.	140	145	19.	152	150
10.	146	140	20.	170	164

points are not exactly on the 45^0 line, they are scattered close to it, suggesting good but not perfect agreement.

Pearson's correlation coefficient (r) calculated from the data is 0.976, indicating a strong correlation between the two measurements. Although Pearson's correlation coefficient is one of the most frequently used measures of agreement, it is *not appropriate* for several reasons, such as: a) the value of r measures the strength of the linear relationship between two measurements, which is not the same as measuring agreement; b) it is possible to get a high degree of correlation between two measurements even when the agreement is poor; c) r is very sensitive to the range of values in the dataset, with data of a higher range yielding a higher r value than data of a lower range; and d) r is also sensitive to extreme values (outliers). Therefore, using the correlation coefficient (r) as a measure of agreement can be misleading [8, 9].

Another common incorrect analysis for agreement is the comparison of means by using a hypothesis test, such as a paired t-test for equality of two means. Even if there is no significant difference in means, we cannot conclude that the two measurements agree well. In our example, the mean difference of systolic BP between two raters is 1.3 mmHg.

12.3.2 Bland-Altman Plot

A Bland-Altman plot is commonly used to describe the agreement between two quantitative measurements. This visual method of assessing agreement does not provide a p-value. It is a scatter plot where the difference between the paired measurements (systolic BP1 – systolic BP2) is plotted on the vertical axis (Y-axis) against the mean of the pair [(systolic BP1 + systolic BP2) ÷ 2] on the horizontal axis (X-axis). Such a plot allows us to easily observe the size of the differences and their distribution around zero (since we expect the difference between two measurements to be zero if they completely agree with each other). Limits of agreement are estimated using (mean difference ± 1.96 x SD) of the differences between the measurements. This plot helps us visually check that the differences are not related to the size of the measurements. If there is good agreement between the measurements, the plot should have the following features: a) the mean difference will be close to zero; b) differences are randomly scattered around zero, with no obvious pattern or trend; and c) data points will be within the limits of agreement (i.e., mean difference ± 1.96 x SD) [3, 7, 10].

We will use the data in Table 12.6 to generate the Bland-Altman plot. Analysis of the data indicates that the mean difference of systolic BP between two raters is 1.3 mmHg, with a standard deviation of 4.8 mmHg. Therefore, the values of (mean difference ± 1.96 x SD) are -8.0 and 10.6, which represent the 95% limits of agreement for the differences.

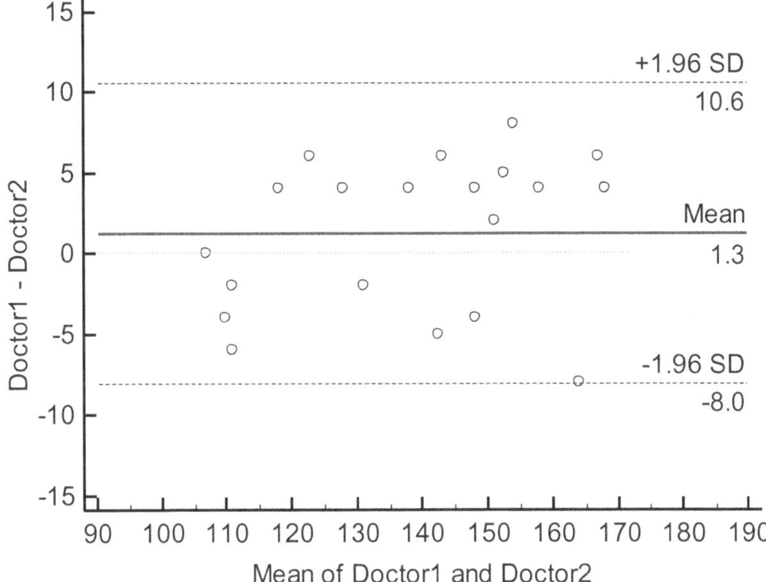

FIGURE 12.2
Bland–Altman plot for systolic blood pressure measured by two doctors.

Figure 12.2 is the Bland-Altman plot generated from the data. The figure shows that the mean difference is 1.3, indicating that, on average, measurements taken by Doctor 1 are slightly higher (by 1.3 mmHg) than measurements taken by Doctor 2. The lower and upper limits of agreement are -8.0 and 10.6, respectively. Ideally, if there is good agreement, the data points should be randomly scattered (without any pattern) around the mean difference line (1.3) and mostly within the limits of agreement (-8.0 to 10.6).

Figure 12.2 shows that all the data points are within the limits of agreement, suggesting there is good agreement between the two doctors' measurements. It also appears from the figure that there is no specific pattern in the differences between two raters' measurements (i.e., the differences did not increase or decrease with the magnitude of the measurements). The mean difference of 1.3 might be considered negligible, depending on the clinical context. The range of the limits of agreement (from -8.0 to 10.6) should be evaluated by the researcher to determine if this range is clinically acceptable for the specific measurement being compared.

In conclusion, the Bland-Altman plot (Figure 12.2) suggests that there is good agreement between Doctor 1 and Doctor 2 for the measurement of systolic BP, with all differences lying within the acceptable range. However, the clinical relevance of the mean difference and the limits of agreement should be judged in the context of the specific application.

12.3.3 Intra-Class Correlation Coefficient

The amount of agreement between continuous variables can be measured quantitatively using the intra-class correlation coefficient (ICC). The ICC is an index of reliability for continuous variables, equivalent to kappa statistics. It indicates the degree of similarity of measurements within groups or classes. It estimates the proportion (fraction) of total measurement variability that is due to variation among individuals. The ICC takes a value between 0 and 1, with 0 indicating no agreement and 1 indicating perfect agreement. In our example (data from Table 12.6), the ICC is 0.986 (calculated by SPSS software), indicating almost perfect agreement of the measurements between doctors [1, 8].

References

1. Ranganathan P, Pramesh CS, Aggarwal R. Common pitfalls in statistical analysis: Measures of agreement. *Perspect Clin Res*. 2017;8(4):187–91. doi:10.4103/picr.PICR_123_17

2. McHugh ML. Interrater reliability: The kappa statistic. *Biochem Med (Zagreb)*. 2012;22(3):276–82. doi:10.11613/BM.2012.031

3. Watson PF, Petrie A. Method agreement analysis: A review of correct methodology. *Theriogenology*. 2010;73(9):1167–79. doi:10.1016/j.theriogenology.2010.01.003

4. Sim J, Wright CC. The kappa statistic in reliability studies: Use, interpretation, and sample size requirements. *Phys Ther*. 2005;85(3):257–68.

5. Viera AJ, Garrett JM. Understanding interobserver agreement: The kappa statistic. *Fam Med*. 2005;37(5):360–3.

6. Landis JR, Koch GG. The measurement of observer agreement for categorical data. *Biometrics*. 1977;33(1):159–74.

7. Altman DG. *Practical Statistics for Medical Research*. 1st ed. New York: Chapman & Hall; 1992.

8. Szklo M, Nieto FJ. *Epidemiology Beyond the Basics*. 2nd ed. Boston: Jones and Bartlett; 2007.

9. Doewes A, Kurdhi NA, Saxena A. Evaluating quadratic weighted kappa as the standard performance metric for automated essay scoring. In: Feng M, Käser T, Talukdar P, eds. *Proceedings of the 16th International Conference on Educational Data Mining*. Bengaluru, India; 2023 Jul:103–13.

10. Chan YH. Biostatistics 104: Correlational analysis. *Singapore Med J*. 2003;44(12):614–9.

13

Investigation of an Epidemic

Mohammad Delwer Hossain Hawlader

Investigating an epidemic is like peeling an onion; layer-by-layer, we uncover the truth hidden within.

Epidemics have been a recurring challenge throughout human history, threatening populations, straining healthcare systems, and causing social and economic disruptions. When faced with the outbreak of a contagious disease, understanding and investigating the epidemic becomes paramount to protect public health and mitigate its impact. This chapter delves into the fascinating world of epidemic investigation, exploring the crucial steps and methods of epidemiologists and public health professionals to unravel the mysteries surrounding the emergence and spread of infectious diseases.

Epidemic investigations serve as a vital tool to protect public health and guide evidence-based decision-making. By studying the dynamics of an outbreak, investigators can develop targeted interventions, implement preventive measures, allocate resources effectively, and inform public health policies. Additionally, these investigations contribute to understanding the disease's natural history, risk factors, and long-term health consequences, laying the foundation for further research and advancements in disease prevention and control.

13.1 Epidemic Investigation

Epidemiologic investigation refers to the systematic and scientific process of studying and analyzing patterns, causes, and effects of health-related events, such as diseases or outbreaks, within a defined population. Epidemic investigations are often referred to as retrospective investigations, as they are frequently conducted after the peak of the epidemic has occurred.

DOI: 10.1201/9781003654803-13

There is no "cookbook" or fixed step-by-step approach that can be universally applied to epidemic investigations, as each investigation is unique and requires tailored methodologies. It is not mandatory to follow all the steps of the investigation process in a specific order. Flexibility is allowed, and investigators can adapt their approach based on the circumstances and available information. It is possible to carry out multiple tasks simultaneously during an epidemic investigation, allowing for efficient use of time and resources. This approach helps expedite the investigation process and facilitates timely decision-making.

13.2 Understanding the Epidemic Landscape

"The first step in solving any problem is recognizing there is one." – Will McAvoy

To effectively combat an epidemic, it is crucial to develop a comprehensive understanding of the epidemic landscape. An epidemic landscape encompasses a wide range of factors, including the disease's dynamics, transmission patterns, affected populations, risk factors, and socio-economic impacts. By delving into the intricacies of this landscape, public health professionals and epidemiologists can gain invaluable insights that inform evidence-based interventions and mitigation strategies.

At the heart of understanding an epidemic landscape lies the analysis of disease dynamics. This involves examining how the disease spreads within and between communities, the rate at which new cases emerge, and the factors influencing its transmission. By analyzing the temporal and spatial patterns of the epidemic, experts can identify hotspots, track its trajectory, and anticipate future trends. Such knowledge is essential for resource allocation, targeted interventions, and early detection of potential outbreaks.

Another critical aspect of understanding an epidemic landscape is identifying the populations most vulnerable to the disease. Factors such as age, gender, pre-existing health conditions, and socio-economic disparities can influence the risk of infection and severity of illness. Analyzing demographic data helps identify high-risk groups, guide public health messaging, and tailor interventions to protect those most susceptible to the disease's adverse effects.

Risk factors play a significant role in shaping the epidemic landscape. These factors can range from behavioral practices and environmental conditions to socio-economic determinants and healthcare access. Investigating and understanding these risk factors provides critical insights into the root causes of the epidemic and guides the development of preventive measures.

By addressing these underlying factors, public health interventions can be designed to effectively mitigate the spread of the disease and reduce its impact on vulnerable populations.

In addition to the scientific aspects, understanding the social and economic impacts of an epidemic is essential. Epidemics have far-reaching consequences, disrupting communities, economies, and healthcare systems. Analyzing the social determinants of health and the economic burden of the epidemic helps policymakers and public health officials assess the wider implications and allocate resources effectively. Understanding the socio-economic landscape enables the development of strategies that not only control the disease but also support affected individuals and communities in their recovery [1].

13.3 Steps of Epidemic Investigation

Epidemic investigation is a vital process in public health that aims to understand the occurrence, spread, and impact of diseases within a population. By following a systematic approach, investigators can identify the root causes, risk factors, and effective control measures to mitigate the effects of an epidemic. The investigation collectively unravels the outbreak's mysteries and guides public health interventions. While the specific details may vary depending on the epidemic's nature, general steps form the foundation of an effective investigation.

Step 1: Verify diagnosis
The initial step in any epidemic investigation is to verify the diagnosis, ensuring the accuracy of reported cases. Trained healthcare professionals assess reported symptoms against clinical criteria to confirm the diagnosis promptly. This confirmation marks the start of a systematic epidemiological investigation involving comprehensive data collection, active surveillance, contact tracing, rigorous data analysis, and laboratory testing. Verifying the diagnosis is crucial to establishing a reliable foundation for understanding disease dynamics, identifying transmission patterns, and developing targeted interventions, ensuring effective epidemic control measures.

Step 2: Confirm the existence of an epidemic
Once the diagnosis is established, the next step is to confirm the existence of an epidemic. An epidemic exists when the number of cases (observed frequency) is more than the expected frequency for that population, based on past experience. An arbitrary limit of two standard deviations (SD) from the endemic occurrence is used to define the epidemic threshold for common

diseases such as flu. Compare with past experience in the same locality (two SD above the mean). Point source epidemics (Hepatitis A virus, cholera, food poisoning) are evident.

Step 3: Define population at risk
To effectively control an epidemic, it is essential to define the population at risk. This step involves identifying the demographic characteristics and geographical locations, and obtaining a map of the area with water collection, residential areas, and a designated number of houses. To count the attack rate, need to use the population censuses for denominator calculation. It should contain information concerning natural landmarks, roads, and the location of dwelling units along each road or in isolated areas. The denominator may be related to the entire population or subgroups of a population. This helps compute the much-needed attack rates in groups or subgroups of the population.

Step 4: Search for causes and their characteristics
Identifying the causes of an epidemic is a critical step in the investigation process. This entails conducting an in-depth analysis to uncover the factors that contribute to disease transmission and outbreak occurrence. Investigations may include:

- Medical survey: Examine the entire population or a subset of the population
- Epidemiological case sheet: Filled for the entire population (sample). It includes:
  - Socio-demographics and socio-economic conditions;
  - History of exposure; and
  - Special event – Sources of the suspected vehicle.
- Concurrently, the medical survey should be carried out in a defined area to identify all, including those who have not sought medical care and those at risk;
- The complete survey will pick all affected individuals with symptoms and signs of the disorder;
- Interview case sheet, designated according to the preliminary rapid inquiry to collect relevant information;
- Name, age, sex, occupation, social class, travel history, history of previous exposure, time of onset of disease, signs and symptoms, personal contact, events as parties, exposure to vehicles as food, water, history of injections, blood products received, etc.;
- Patient will be asked if they know other cases at home, work, neighborhood, or school;

- Search for new cases (secondary cases) should be done every day till the area is declared free of the epidemic; and
- This search period should be twice the incubation period of the disease since the occurrence of the last case.

Step 5: Data analysis
Data analysis is a fundamental component of the epidemic investigation. It involves collecting, organizing, and analyzing relevant data to discern patterns, trends, and associations. Statistical methods, modelling techniques, and visualization tools are used to extract meaningful insights from the data, aiding in the understanding of disease dynamics and informing intervention strategies. During data analysis, the following points should be taken into consideration:

- Person's characteristics: Age, sex, occupation, exposure to a specific event;
- Place (spot map): To show clustering of cases (common source) – to provide evidence of source and mode of spread, like John Snow in the cholera outbreak in London;
- Determine the attack rates/case fatality rates for exposed and non-exposed, and according to host factors;
- Time (epidemic curve): An epidemic curve suggests the following:
  - A time relationship with exposure to a suspected source;
  - Whether it is a common source or a propagated epidemic; and
  - Whether it is a seasonal or cyclic pattern suggestive of a particular infection.

Step 6: Hypothesis formulation
Based on the data analysis, investigators formulate hypotheses to explain the observed patterns and associations. These hypotheses serve as the foundation for further investigation and guide the design of studies or experiments aimed at testing their validity. Hypothesis formulation allows for a focused approach to uncovering the underlying factors driving the epidemic. On the basis of agent-host-environment, formulate a hypothesis to explain the epidemic in terms of:

- Possible source;
- Causative agent;
- Possible modes of spread; and
- Predisposing environmental factors.

Step 7: Testing the hypothesis
The next step involves testing the formulated hypotheses through rigorous scientific methods. This may include conducting controlled studies, field investigations, or experiments to gather additional evidence and assess the validity of the hypotheses. All reasonable hypotheses need to be considered and weighed by comparing attack rates in various groups for those exposed and non-exposed to each suspected factor. Consider and test alternative hypotheses to find which hypothesis is consistent with all the facts.

Step 8: Evaluation of ecological factors
In many epidemics, ecological factors play a significant role in disease transmission and outbreak dynamics. An epidemiologist's concern is to relate the disease to environmental factors to know the source, reservoir, and modes of transmission. Possible ecological factors to investigate include: a) Sanitation status; b) Water supply; c) Population movement; d) Atmospheric changes, such as temperature, humidity, and air pollution; and e) Population dynamics of vectors and animal reservoirs. Assessing these ecological factors helps in identifying potential interventions and preventive measures targeting the underlying causes.

Step 9: Further investigation of at-risk factors
Once the initial investigations are conducted, it is important to delve deeper into specific risk factors associated with the epidemic. This may involve:

- Prospective or retrospective collection of additional information through clinical examination, screening test, examination of food, stool, or blood specimen, and biochemical studies; and
- Detect sub-clinical cases and classify the population according to exposure and illness status into exposure to a specific potential vehicle and whether ill or not.

Step 10: Report writing
The final step in the epidemic investigation is the compilation and dissemination of findings through a comprehensive report. This report summarizes the following:

- Background of the investigation;
- Geographical location;
  - Climate condition;
  - Demographic status (population pyramid);
  - Socioeconomic status;
  - Organization of health services;
  - Surveillance and early warning systems;

- Normal disease pattern;
- Historical data;
- Methods of investigation;
- Data analysis;
- Significance of results; and
- Preventive recommendation.

13.4 Historical Evidence of Epidemic Investigation

13.4.1 Broad Street Cholera Outbreak (1854)

Dr John Snow's investigation of the Broad Street cholera outbreak in London stands as a landmark event in the epidemic investigation. Snow's meticulous research and mapping of cases led him to identify contaminated water from a public pump as the source of the cholera outbreak. This investigation laid the foundation for recognizing the role of contaminated water in transmitting cholera and revolutionizing sanitation practices [2].

13.4.2 Spanish Flu Pandemic (1918–1919)

The investigation of the Spanish flu pandemic offered valuable insights into the epidemiology of a global influenza outbreak. Epidemiologists and researchers conducted extensive investigations to understand risk factors, transmission patterns, and the impact of the virus. These investigations helped shape future pandemic response strategies and influenced public health measures for managing respiratory diseases [3].

13.4.3 SARS Outbreak (2002–2003)

The investigation of the severe acute respiratory syndrome (SARS) outbreak exemplifies international collaboration and rapid response in epidemic investigations. Epidemiologists worked across borders to study transmission dynamics, identify the SARS-CoV virus, and implement control measures. The lessons learned from this investigation influenced subsequent efforts to combat emerging infectious diseases and strengthen global surveillance systems [4].

13.4.4 Ebola Outbreak in West Africa (2014–2016)

The investigation of the Ebola virus outbreak in Guinea, Liberia, and Sierra Leone highlights the challenges of investigating highly contagious and deadly diseases. Epidemiologists and public health experts played pivotal roles in tracing contacts, implementing quarantine measures, and developing treatment and prevention strategies. This investigation significantly advanced our understanding of Ebola transmission dynamics and informed subsequent outbreak response efforts [5].

13.4.5 Outbreak of COVID-19 (2019–2022)

COVID-19, caused by SARS-CoV-2, has become a pandemic worldwide in a very short span of time. The outbreak started in Wuhan City, China, and spread to almost all parts of the world, and is considered one of the most serious pandemic diseases in the world. The high transmission rate and pathogenicity of this virus have made COVID-19 a major public health concern globally. Basically, the emergence of SARS-CoV-2 is the third introduction of a highly infectious human epidemic coronavirus in the twenty-first century. Investigations of SARS-CoV-2 have been conducted by various research groups and have claimed bats to be the natural host of SARS-CoV-2. COVID-19 cost hundreds of thousands of lives, and millions faced the consequences.

In conclusion, investigation of an epidemic involves a comprehensive exploration of etiology, transmission patterns, and control measures. Collaboration among epidemiologists, healthcare professionals, and communities is crucial for gathering vital data and utilizing advanced technologies to detect and identify outbreaks swiftly. Rigorous analysis of collected data provides insights into the disease's etiology, risk factors, and impact. Modelling and simulation aid in projecting future trends and guiding effective public health interventions. Challenges such as information dissemination, balancing public health measures with individual rights, and addressing social determinants of health persist. Our commitment to knowledge, collaboration, and resilience is essential in mitigating the impact of epidemics and creating a healthier and more equitable world.

References

1. Pendergrast M. *Inside the Outbreaks: The Elite Medical Detectives of the Epidemic Intelligence Service*. 2010;16(7):1188. doi:10.3201/eid1607.100582
2. Metcalfe C. *The Ghost Map*. Steven Johnson. *Int J Epidemiol*. 2007;36(4):935–36. doi:10.1093/IJE/DYM111
3. Barry JM. *The Great Influenza: The Epic Story of the Deadliest Plague in History*. New York: Viking Press; 2004. www.jci.org.
4. Lee SH. The SARS epidemic in Hong Kong: What lessons have we learned? *J R Soc Med*. 2003;96(8):374. doi:10.1258/JRSM.96.8.374
5. Jacob ST, Crozier I, Fischer WA, Hewlett A, Kraft CS, Vega MA de L, et al. Ebola virus disease. *Nat Rev Dis Primers*. 2020;6(1):13. doi:10.1038/S41572-020-0147-3

14

Public Health Surveillance

Russell Kabir

The term "surveillance" has come from the French words "sur", which means over, and "veiller", which means to watch [1]. According to the World Health Organization (WHO) [2], "surveillance is the ongoing systematic collection, analysis, and interpretation of health data". Hence, it can be said that "public health surveillance is the ongoing collection, analysis, and dissemination of health-related data to provide information that can be used to monitor and improve the health of populations" [3].

The key objectives of public health surveillance are: a) explore information on the changing trends in the health status of the population using indicators such as mortality, morbidity, nutritional status, obesity rate, pollution level, or accessibility of services that have direct or indirect impact on health; b) data from the surveillance system helps to shape up the policy, improves the effectiveness and efficiency of health system and services by identifying the gaps in the services; and c) finally, it is used as a useful tool for providing early warning sign of any public health disasters so early interventions can be introduced to reduce the causalities and further risks.

Public Health surveillance was primarily focused on infectious diseases. Still, in recent times it has been used for monitoring injuries, pregnancy complications and congenital disabilities, chronic diseases, and environmental risk factors such as physical, chemical, biological, or psychosocial, and health behaviors of the population [4].

The key elements of the surveillance are: a) identification of the health problem; b) collection of existing data to monitor the progress of the health problem; c) analysis and summarization of data and preparation of a report based on the findings; and d) finally, sharing the report with the health authorities to develop policy (Figure 14.1).

DOI: 10.1201/9781003654803-14

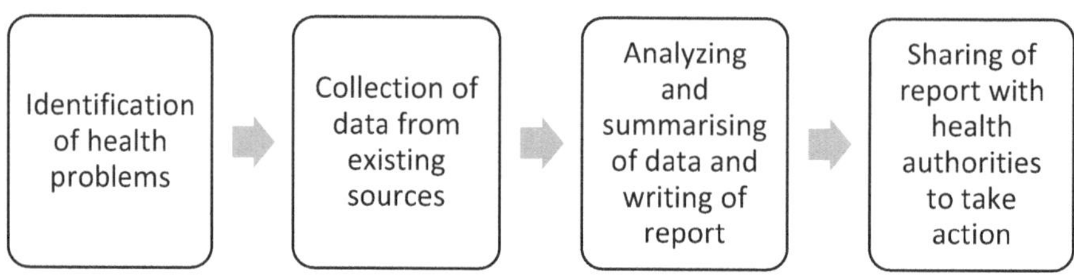

FIGURE 14.1
Key elements of the surveillance system. (Adapted from Macera et al. [5].)

14.1 Uses of Public Health Surveillance

Public health surveillance helps to:

- Estimate the magnitude of a health problem or disease;
- Detect epidemics or define a problem;
- Identification of disease in terms of time, place, and person;
- Depict the natural history of a disease;
- To detect changes in health practices;
- Expedite emergency planning when there is an outbreak;
- Monitor changes in infectious agents; and
- Early identification of risk factors of a disease can be used to predict future disease occurrence.

14.2 Components of Surveillance

Surveillance plays a crucial role in identifying disease outbreaks, monitoring trends in health conditions, assessing the impact of interventions, and guiding public health actions. The components of public health surveillance include:

Data Collection: Detailed but necessary data are collected from the target group. The data collection process should specify what is to be reported, by whom, how to report, and how often. This involves the systematic and ongoing collection of data from the identified sources. Data can be collected through different methods, such as case reporting, laboratory testing, surveys, and syndromic surveillance, etc.

Compilation and analysis: Collected data must be analyzed to identify trends, patterns, and potential public health threats. Epidemiologists and other public health professionals analyze the data to detect outbreaks, track disease spread, and assess the effectiveness of interventions.

Interpretation: Data interpretation involves making sense of the analyzed data to understand the implications for public health. This step helps identify health risks, vulnerable populations, and areas that require targeted interventions. Similarities between current and past situations and similarities or dissimilarities with other populations.

Dissemination: Surveillance data needs to be shared with key stakeholders, such as public health officials, healthcare providers, policymakers, and the general public. Timely and accurate dissemination of information helps inform decision-making and public health actions.

14.3 Types of Surveillance

Public health surveillance encompasses various approaches to monitor and track health-related data to protect and promote public health. Different types of public health surveillance methods are discussed below [5].

14.3.1 Active Surveillance

In an active surveillance system, healthcare workers are hired to go out regularly to healthcare providers and facilities, including hospitals, clinics, and primary healthcare centers, to look for newly diagnosed cases of the disease, existing cases of the disease, or fatalities caused by the disease. Identifying newly diagnosed cases of disease, existing cases of disease, or fatalities is known as case finding [6]. It is typically used to gather data about rare diseases that could have a considerable impact on public health, such as meningococcal infections or severe acute respiratory syndrome (SARS), or when cases need to be followed up with public health intervention, such as immunization, quarantine, chemoprophylaxis, and contact tracing. With the active surveillance system, public health professionals can collect more detailed data, and this system provides improved sensitivity. On the other hand, this is an expensive and time-consuming process [7].

14.3.2 Passive Surveillance

In passive surveillance, public health professionals use the available data on diseases or health conditions. Public health professionals regularly monitor and report cases without active involvement in identification and reporting. The health care provider must report the disease or health condition status. This type of reporting is called passive reporting; hence, the accuracy and reliability of the reported data are highly dependent on the individual. Therefore, inadequate and incomplete reporting is likely to occur, but this is not a costly method and is easy to develop. An example of passive surveillance is when an elderly care home reports an unusual number of elderly patients with unexplained skin rashes.

14.3.3 Syndromic Surveillance

In syndromic surveillance, clinical information about disease signs and symptoms is collected before a diagnosis is made, and generally uses electronic data from hospital emergency rooms. An example of syndromic surveillance is hospital admittance records. This is very useful to monitor seasonal disease trends, identify outbreaks, and provide information on sudden and unexpected changes in disease trends. The advantage of syndromic surveillance is the early detection of any abnormalities within a short time. In addition to collecting medical records on the syndrome, it thoroughly uses additional data sources, including drug sales, laboratory results, medical examinations, records of ambulance calls, absences from school or the workplace, and additional symptoms and signs in emergency rescue [8]. The key limitation of this system is a lack of specificity.

14.3.4 Sentinel Surveillance

When high-quality data cannot be collected through a passive surveillance system, a sentinel surveillance system is used. The Sentinel surveillance system provides the opportunity to focus on specific regions to gather information about risk across wider study areas, lowering the number of resources needed by restricting the number of sample units and effort. It is designed to collect data that will aid in the identification of crucial public health issues and the development of effective prevention and control measures at the local and national levels, aid in the monitoring and assessment of current prevention and control measures, and promote the growth of a public health network that encompasses epidemiological and laboratory expertise. It is unsuitable for detecting rare diseases and requires more time and resources than passive surveillance. However, well-designed sentinel surveillance can rapidly identify outbreaks. For example, public health professionals in Canada use a sentinel surveillance system to monitor influenza activity [7, 9].

14.3.5 Behavioral Surveillance

This kind of surveillance system identifies risk factors and collects data on any trait, characteristics or exposure that increases the risk of developing an infection, illness or injury. Accurate behavioral data helps as an early warning system, and public health professionals can arrange the best resources in a timely manner to keep the prevalence level low. Also, tracking behaviors over time provides a substantially more sensitive indicator of the success of national program initiatives. Sometimes, a lack of behavioral data can slow the process of outbreak control. For example, behavioral surveillance helps track sexually transmitted infectious diseases such as HIV/AIDS [10].

14.4 Steps of Public Health Surveillance

The steps for conducting public health surveillance are as follows:

- *Establish objectives:* While planning a surveillance system, it is essential to set clear objectives before data collection. For example, a surveillance team can develop objectives to assess the public health status, evaluate public health programs, or conduct research.

- *Develop case definitions:* The criteria to define a case of the disease or health event need to be decided. This will ensure accurate and consistent data collection.

- *Determine data sources:* Generally, the data is collected from medical records, laboratory reports, regional or national statistical offices, and self-reported survey data.

- *Determine data-collection methods:* This can be done using active, passive, sentinel, syndromic, or behavioral surveillance systems.

- *Field-test methods:* Once the data collection method is confirmed, the data to be collected by a surveillance system, the data sources and collection methods, and the procedures for handling the information should be developed and tested.

- *Develop and test analytic approach:* Using appropriate statistical tests, data is analyzed to identify trends, patterns, and potential public health issues.

- *Interpretation and dissemination:* Decision-makers at all levels can easily understand and comprehend the implications of the information; data must be accurately analyzed and presented. Public health specialists and healthcare workers are the primary recipients of surveillance data. The analysis, interpretations, and recommendations from the surveillance data should be included in information aimed primarily at those people.

- *Evaluation:* The surveillance system should be periodically evaluated to assess its effectiveness and efficiency. This evaluation helps identify potential weaknesses and opportunities for improvement [11].

14.5 Ways to Improve Surveillance

Improving public health surveillance is essential to enhance the early detection and response to health threats, monitor health trends, and guide effective public health interventions. Here are some ways to improve public health surveillance:

Expand the scope of surveillance: Traditional public health surveillance systems have focused on infectious diseases. However, there is a growing need to expand surveillance to include chronic diseases, mental health conditions, and other health threats.

Improve data quality: The quality of data is essential for accurate public health surveillance. Public health agencies need to invest in quality assurance programs to ensure that data is collected and reported accurately.

Make data more accessible: Public health data should be made more accessible to researchers, public health practitioners, and the public. This will help to improve the understanding of health trends and the development of effective public health interventions.

Improve awareness of the provider and recipients: Persons collecting data must be aware of the responsibility. The persons must know the conditions to be reported. Similarly, the recipients should have an awareness of better data collection.

Training to the providers: Train a workforce with the skills needed for public health surveillance. Public health agencies need to train a workforce with the skills needed to collect, analyze, and interpret health data. This includes epidemiologists, data scientists, and information technology professionals.

Make data-driven decisions: Public health agencies should use data to make decisions about public health interventions. This includes decisions about how to allocate resources, what policies to implement, and how to communicate with the public.

Targeted surveillance: Implement targeted surveillance for specific high-risk populations or regions to monitor diseases that disproportionately affect certain groups. This approach can lead to more effective and tailored interventions.

Data analytics and machine learning: Utilize advanced data analytics and machine learning algorithms to analyze large datasets, identify patterns, and predict disease trends. These technologies can provide valuable insights for decision-making.

Global health collaboration: Engage in international collaborations and data sharing to respond to global health challenges effectively. Infectious diseases often cross borders, making global cooperation crucial.

References

1. Chan KC. The past, present, and future of public health surveillance. *Scientifica*. 2012;2012:875253. doi:10.6064/2012/875253.
2. World Health Organization. *Public Health Surveillance*; 2023. Available from: www.afro.who.int/health-topics/public-health-surveillance.
3. Soucie JM. Public health surveillance and data collection: General principles and impact on hemophilia care. *Hematology*. 2012;17(Suppl 1):S144–6.
4. Merrill RM. *Introduction to Epidemiology*. 7th ed. Burlington, MA: Jones & Bartlett Learning; 2019.
5. Macera CA, Shaffer R, Shaffer PM. *Introduction to Epidemiology: Distribution and Determinants of Disease*. New York: Cengage Learning; 2013.
6. Gordis L. *Epidemiology*. 5th ed. Philadelphia, PA: Elsevier Health Sciences; 2013.
7. Gilbert R, Cliffe SJ. Public health surveillance. In: Regmi K, Gee I. (eds) *Public Health Intelligence*. Cham: Springer; 2016:91–110.
8. Yang W. *Early Warning for Infectious Disease Outbreak: Theory and Practice*. London, UK: Academic Press; 2017.
9. Anderson C. Sentinel health unit surveillance system. *Can J Infect Dis*. 1994;5(5):207–9.
10. Brown T. Behavioral surveillance: Current perspectives, and its role in catalyzing action. *J Acquir Immune Defic Syndr*. 2003;32(Suppl 1):S12–7. doi:10.1097/00126334-200302011-00003
11. Teutsch SM, Thacker SB. Planning a public health surveillance system. *Epidemiol Bull*. 1995;16(1):1–6.

15

Bias, Confounding, and Interaction in Epidemiological Studies

Mohammad Tajul Islam

Bias, in addition to confounding, is a major concern in all kinds of epidemiological studies, especially observational study designs. The presence of bias in a study affects its internal validity.

Validity (also see Chapter 11) in research refers to how well a study measures what it is supposed to measure and whether the conclusions drawn from the study are accurate and reliable. Validity of study results is essential for ensuring the usefulness of research findings. It is broadly categorized into internal validity and external validity.

Internal validity examines whether the design, execution, and analysis of a study are reliable enough to produce trustworthy answers to the research questions. If a study is free from biases or confounding factors, it has internal validity and provides a correct association between exposure and outcome. Therefore, achieving high internal validity is essential for drawing meaningful conclusions about a study's results.

External validity, or generalizability, is the applicability of the study results obtained in one study population to other populations [1]. For example, if a study conducted in a white population finds an association between coffee consumption and stomach cancer, and the results are also applicable to a non-white population, the study is said to have external validity. There is no external validity if the study does not have internal validity. Therefore, ensuring internal validity of a study should always be the primary objective.

Bias is a systematic error resulting from flaws either in the study design, the method of selection of study subjects, or the procedure of collecting information related to exposure and/or outcome. If bias is present, the study results tend to be different from the true results. For example, due to bias, a case-control study may report an odds ratio (OR) of 2.0 for a certain association, even though no association exists in the population.

DOI: 10.1201/9781003654803-15

Bias can be defined as "any systematic error in an epidemiological study that results in an incorrect estimate of the association between exposure and the risk of disease" [2]. Simply, a study is said to be biased if the study result is different from the true value. If the design and procedure of a study are unbiased, the study is considered valid.

There is another type of error, called random error, which needs to be distinguished from systematic error or bias (also see Section 16.1). Random error affects precision and produces a wide confidence interval. Random error is directly related to the sample size of the study [1, 3]. Random error results from the use of sample values to estimate the population parameters in the reference population. When the sample size is small, the sample estimate may differ substantially from the population value due to random error. Random error cannot be completely eliminated, but it can be minimized by taking a large sample from the population.

Bias is a major concern in epidemiological studies, as it can distort the true association between exposures and outcomes, leading to incorrect conclusions about the study findings. Controlling for bias is essential to ensure the validity and reliability of study findings, which help in public health decision-making. In general, bias in a study can be prevented or controlled by a) selecting an appropriate study design to address the hypothesis; b) careful monitoring of data collection to ensure that the data are valid and reliable; and c) using appropriate analytic procedures [3].

Systematic errors or biases can be broadly classified into *selection bias and information (or observation) bias*. There is another type of bias, called *confounding bias,* that should also be considered when designing a study and analyzing the data [1–6].

15.1 Selection Bias

Selection bias occurs if the study result is affected by the faulty process of selecting cases or controls, or exposed or unexposed groups. Selection bias commonly occurs when a non-comparable group is selected as the comparison group, especially in case-control studies.

When individuals with exposure (or outcome) have different probabilities of being selected compared to those not selected in a study, selection bias is likely to occur. Such a bias can occur when exposed cases have a higher probability of being selected in a case-control study. An example of this type of bias is the *surveillance bias, also known as detection bias or ascertainment bias.*

Surveillance bias occurs when subjects in the exposed group under surveillance are more likely to have the study outcome detected. For example, suppose a cohort study was conducted to determine the association between

TABLE 15.1

A case-control study data from the whole population

	Case	Control
Exposed	500	2,000
Unexposed	500	7,000
Total	**1,000**	**9,000**

Odds ratio (OR) = 3.5

TABLE 15.2

Data with a 50% sample from cases and a 10% sample from controls

	Case	Control
Exposed	250	200
Unexposed	250	700
Total	**500**	**900**

Odds ratio (OR) = 3.5

oral contraceptive (OC) use and cervical cancer, using surveillance data for OC users as the exposed group and non-surveillance data for those who did not use OC. Because of the surveillance of OC users, it is more likely that cervical cancer cases at an early stage will be identified at a higher rate due to regular screening than in non-users of OC. As a result, the study may demonstrate an overestimation of the association between OC use and cervical cancer.

Let us see how selection bias occurs in a study when the exposure rate in cases (or controls) is different from the population. Here, we present the data of a hypothetical case-control study, assuming that the study is free from other kinds of biases (information or confounding bias). Table 15.1 shows the number of cases and controls by exposure status in a population of 10,000 people. The proportion exposed among cases is 50.0% (500 ÷ 1,000), and that among controls is 22.2% (2,000 ÷ 9,000). The calculated odds ratio (OR) is 3.5.

Now, let us take a 50% sample of cases and a 10% sample of controls from the population, as shown in Table 15.2. The proportion of cases exposed (50.0%) and the proportion of controls exposed (22.2%) remain the same as in the population (Table 15.1). The calculated OR is 3.5, which is the same as the population OR. This indicates that as long as the exposure rate in cases and the exposure rate in controls remain unchanged during the selection process, the OR will remain the same (unbiased).

TABLE 15.3

Data with a 50% sample from cases and a 10% sample from controls

	Case	Control
Exposed	350	200
Unexposed	150	700
Total	**500**	**900**

Odds ratio (OR) = 8.2

However, the situation will be different if the proportion exposed among cases (or controls) is affected by the way samples are selected, as shown in Table 15.3. The table shows that even though 50% of cases and 10% of controls are selected from the population, the proportion of cases exposed is 70.0%, which is higher than the exposure rate among cases in the population (i.e., the selection of cases is not independent). The calculated OR is 8.3, which is higher than the actual value of 3.5. This example illustrates how selection bias can occur in a study.

It is important to note that such consequences are unintentional, and the researcher may not be aware of such a phenomenon. In reality, a complete list of cases occurring in a population is not available. Researchers often use convenience sampling to select both cases and controls, such as selecting cases and controls from hospitals, making the occurrence of the selection bias more likely. Selection bias occurring in hospital-based case-control studies (when the probability of hospitalization of cases and controls differs) is often referred to as *Berksonian bias.*

Selection bias may occur if the eligibility criteria for cases and controls are different. The bias resulting from such differences is known as *exclusion bias.* For example, a hospital-based case-control study was conducted to find an association between the use of reserpine (an antihypertensive drug) and breast cancer. The investigators selected women without breast cancer as controls from the surgery department after excluding those who were operated on for conditions such as cholecystectomy, thyroidectomy, surgery for renal disease, and any cardiac operations, as they were more likely to have used reserpine. The investigators were concerned that if these conditions were not excluded from the control group, it might artificially increase the exposure rate in the control group, and the association may be diluted. However, the investigators did not exclude these conditions while selecting cases (women with breast cancer). As a result, a positive association was found between the use of reserpine and breast cancer. Studies conducted subsequently, excluding these conditions from both cases and controls, did not find any association [3].

Non-response and individuals lost to follow-up can also introduce selection bias in a study when participants differ from non-participants or those lost to follow-up. It may be difficult to assess the bias since no information is available from the non-respondents or those lost to follow-up. Studies show that people who respond (participate) in a study are often different from those who do not respond in terms of demographic, socio-economic, cultural, lifestyle, and other characteristics. Similarly, individuals lost to follow-up may also differ from those who remain in the study until the occurrence of an event or the termination of the study. It is, therefore, important to keep the non-response and loss to follow-up as minimal as possible in a study [1, 3].

In cohort studies, selection bias is less likely to occur because study subjects are selected before the development of an outcome. Nevertheless, selection bias may occur at the outset of a cohort study while selecting the exposed or unexposed group. For example, in occupational cohort studies, bias may be introduced when mortality or morbidity rates in the occupationally exposed group are compared with the general population (*healthy worker effect*) [1]. The reason is that individuals in an occupation need to remain healthy in order to be in the job. Ill and unhealthy people are usually excluded from this group, while the general population includes both healthy and unhealthy individuals, making the comparison inappropriate. As a result, the morbidity and mortality rates in the occupational group are likely to be lower than in the general population, which is referred to as the *healthy worker effect*.

15.2 Information Bias

Information bias occurs when the means of obtaining information from study subjects are inadequate. Information bias arises because of the use of imperfect definitions of variables (such as exposure or outcome) or faulty data collection procedures. This may result in *misclassification bias* (misclassification of cases or of exposure) and *recall bias* [1–4].

Misclassification of cases (or controls) occurs due to the inaccuracy (because of varying sensitivity and specificity; see Chapter 11) of the diagnostic test. Because of misclassification, a diseased person may be classified as non-diseased and vice versa. Similarly, misclassification of exposure may occur due to inaccuracies in the record-keeping system, which may classify exposed persons as unexposed and vice versa. Misclassification can be of two types: a) *differential misclassification* and b) *non-differential misclassification*.

In differential misclassification, the degree (or proportion) of misclassification (of exposure or outcome) differs between the groups being compared. For example, in a case-control study, there is a 10% misclassification of exposure among cases and a 15% misclassification of exposure among controls (or a

10% misclassification of cases and a 15% misclassification of controls among exposed and unexposed groups, respectively). In differential misclassification, the risk estimate is biased either toward or away from the null value, depending on the proportion of subjects misclassified.

In non-differential misclassification, the proportion of misclassification (of exposure or outcome) is the same across the groups being compared. For example, exposure is equally misclassified (e.g., 10%) in both cases and controls (i.e., the same proportion of exposure is misclassified in both groups). In non-differential misclassification, the risk estimate is biased toward the null value.

Recall bias occurs due to the inability of study participants to remember past events (exposures) equally among cases and controls. In other words, recall bias occurs when the presence of disease leads to a better recall of past exposure. For example, in a case-control study, cases may be more likely to remember a past exposure than controls if the exposure is widely known to be associated with the disease under investigation.

Recall bias is more common in case-control studies, in which participants already know their disease status. For example, in a case-control study examining rubella infection during pregnancy as a risk factor for congenital heart disease in newborns, mothers who gave birth to babies with congenital heart disease may be more likely to remember a rubella infection during pregnancy than mothers who gave birth to babies without heart disease.

Interviewer bias is another type of information bias. Interviewer bias arises when an interviewer consciously or unconsciously collects inaccurate information from study subjects. This may happen when the interviewer (or the data collector) is aware of the outcome (or exposure) status of an individual and the hypothesis to be tested in the study. For example, in a case-control study, if the interviewer knew the outcome status of an individual, s/he might probe more deeply for evidence of exposure among cases than among controls. Interviewer bias may also occur in cohort studies (or clinical trials) when an interviewer tries to elicit evidence of the outcome more meticulously in exposed than in unexposed subjects.

Another potential source of information bias in epidemiological studies is the *Hawthorne effect*, also known as the *observer effect*. The Hawthorne effect refers to the tendency of individuals to change their behavior when they become aware that they are being observed. As a result, the observed behavior may not reflect the "normal" behavior of individuals, which may affect the validity of the study findings. For example, in a study on infection prevention at healthcare settings, hospital staff may adopt more frequent handwashing practices when they are aware that they are being observed. The Hawthorne effect can be mitigated by blinding the subjects, where participants will not know that they are being observed. Moreover, observing participants over an extended period of time can help minimize the Hawthorne effect, as participants are likely to become accustomed to being observed and revert to their normal behavior.

15.3 Confounding

Confounding is another type of bias important in epidemiological studies. Confounding, if present in a study, can cause an overestimation or underestimation of the actual association between exposure and disease. Bias introduced by a confounding factor can be large, and it can even change the apparent direction of an effect. Confounding bias is more likely to occur in observational studies than in randomized experimental studies. However, unlike selection and information bias, it can be adjusted during data analysis.

15.3.1 What Is Confounding?

When the strength of association [odds ratio (OR) or relative risk (RR)] between an exposure and the outcome of interest is changed due to the presence of a third variable (factor), the phenomenon is called confounding, and the third variable is called the confounding factor or confounding variable. Confounding is a common occurrence in etiological studies, since mostly multiple factors are associated with disease rather than a single factor. If there is only one factor causing the disease, confounding is not possible.

Confounding can be present by nature in any study (e.g., cohort, case-control, cross-sectional, or ecological studies). It is not primarily due to the study design. Of all study designs, ecological studies are most susceptible to confounding bias and are difficult to control because of the use of aggregated data. In all other study designs, as long as there is available data on potential confounders, they can be adjusted during analysis. Confounding should be of concern in the following situations [3]:

When evaluating an exposure-disease association: Confounding is always a concern when claiming that an exposure is causally associated with an outcome. To explicitly express such a relationship, it is essential to ensure that the association is free from the influence of other factors.

Quantifying the degree of association between an exposure and disease: For example, an investigator is interested in quantifying the risk of heart disease in diabetes. When a precise estimate of the risk is the goal, adjusting for confounding factors is imperative. In one study, an RR of four may decrease to 3.6 after controlling for confounding factors, while in another study, it may change to 1.2 or even exceed four after adjusting for confounders.

Multiple causal pathways may lead to the disease: If there is only one factor associated with the disease, confounding is not possible. Multiple factors are virtually always associated with the causation of a disease. It is therefore necessary to control other factors to quantify the risk of a factor of interest. For example, when evaluating the risk of heart disease associated with being overweight, the association should be adjusted for factors such as serum cholesterol level, hypertension, diabetes, and other factors that may influence the relationship between being overweight and heart disease.

Each potential confounding factor (variable) has to meet two criteria. They include: a) the confounding variable must be causally associated with the disease of interest, i.e., it must be a risk factor for the disease independently; and b) the distribution of the confounding variable should be different in exposed and unexposed groups under investigation, i.e., the proportion of the confounding factor among exposed and unexposed groups should be different (in other words, the confounding factor is causally or non-causally associated with the exposure of interest).

For instance, in a study to evaluate whether hypertension is a cause of heart disease, diabetes should be considered a confounding factor if a) diabetes is a known risk factor for heart disease; and b) diabetes is associated with hypertension (exposure of interest), but it is not a consequence of hypertension (Figure 15.1).

All potential confounding factors should be independently associated with the disease under investigation, but they should not be part of the proposed exposure-disease pathway. For instance, if someone is interested in evaluating the association between maternal undernutrition and low birthweight, anemia should not be counted as a confounding factor if it is considered an intermediary step in the causal pathway between maternal undernutrition and low birthweight (Figure 15.2). However, if the proposed causal pathway is independent of anemia, then anemia should be considered a potential confounder.

15.3.2 Types of Confounding Effects

The presence of a confounding factor may cause an overestimation or underestimation of the true strength of the association. A confounding factor can

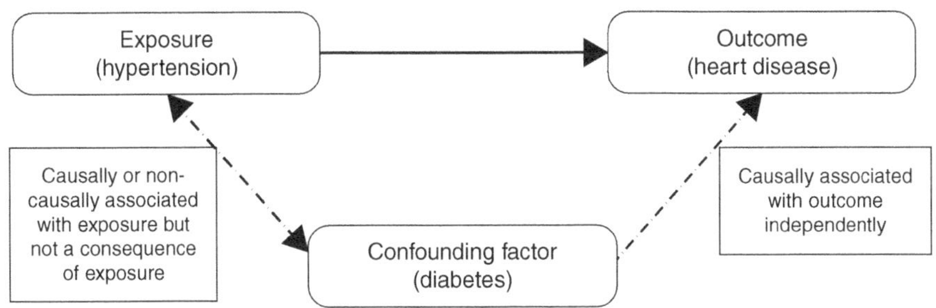

FIGURE 15.1

Interrelationship between exposure, confounding factor, and outcome.

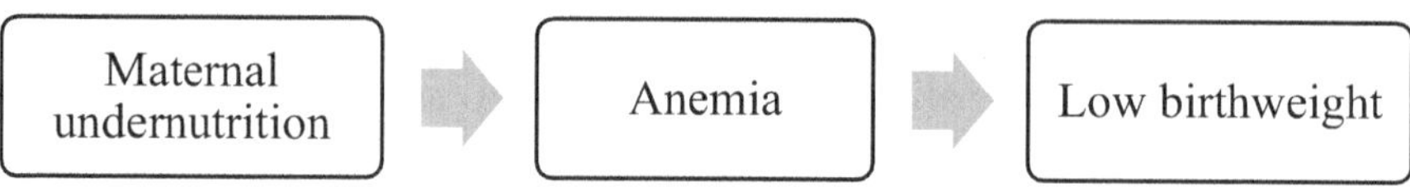

FIGURE 15.2

Interrelationship between an exposure (maternal undernutrition), an outcome (low birthweight), and a potential confounding factor (anemia).

Notes: If the factor "anemia" is in the causal pathway between maternal undernutrition and low birthweight, it should not be considered a confounding factor

have the following effects on the strength of the association between an exposure and an outcome.

Positive confounding: Positive confounding occurs when the measure of risk (RR or OR) is greater than the actual value in the presence of one or more confounding factors. In positive confounding, the measure of risk will decrease after adjustment. For example, the crude RR of lung cancer for smoking is calculated as 3.5, but when adjusted for sex, it is found to be 2.5. Here, the confounding factor "sex" has a positive confounding effect.

Negative confounding: Negative confounding occurs when the presence of a confounding factor reduces the measure of risk of an exposure on the outcome, so that the magnitude of risk increases after adjustment. For example, the crude RR of lung cancer for smoking is 2.5 in a study, but when adjusted for age, it is found to be 3.5.

Qualitative confounding: When the relationship (risk estimate) is reversed after adjustment (reciprocal relationship), it is called qualitative confounding. For example, in a study, the crude RR of cervical cancer for human papillomavirus infection is found to be 0.7. However, when adjusted for the number of sexual partners, it is found to be 1.8.

15.3.3 Control of Confounding Factors

Once the actual confounding factors have been identified in a study, the next step is to adjust for these confounding effects to obtain the true estimate of the association. Depending on the number of confounding factors, there are various ways to adjust them. Confounding factors can be adjusted both during the design and analysis phases of a study. During the design phase, the confounding factors can be controlled by:

Randomization: Randomization, or random allocation, is possible in experimental studies such as clinical trials and community trials. Randomization is the process of randomly allocating interventions to study groups (see Section 9.8). Randomization makes study groups identical in terms of known and unknown factors, provided the sample size is sufficiently large. It is therefore an effective way of controlling the confounding factors.

Restriction: A confounding factor(s) can be controlled in a study by restricting study participants to those without the confounding factor. For example, excluding individuals with diabetes (a confounding factor) in a study evaluating the relationship between hypertension and heart disease. While restrictions do not affect the internal validity, they may limit the generalizability of the study's findings.

Matching: Matching, when done on one or more confounding variables, is an effective way of controlling confounding factors in a study, provided the data are analyzed with the matched pair design (e.g., using conditional logistic regression analysis). Matching is primarily used in case-control studies. In a matched design, cases and controls are paired based on one or more potential confounding factors, ensuring that the distribution of factors matched is identical across groups. Matching, however, does not control the factors for which matching is not done.

During data analysis, whenever a confounding factor(s) is identified in a study, it is necessary to control it to obtain the actual effect of exposure on the outcome. Fortunately, confounding factors can be adjusted during data analysis, and there are three ways to adjust them:

Restricting the analysis: In this strategy, data are analyzed for the association between exposure and disease at one level (category) of the confounding factor. For example, if sex is a confounding factor in the relationship between chewing betel quid and oral cancer, analyze the data only for males or females. The problem with this approach is that we end up with a smaller sample size, throwing up a big chunk of data.

Stratified analysis: Stratified analysis is suitable for the adjustment of one or two confounding factors. In stratified analysis, the crude measure of association is compared with the adjusted measure of association to assess the confounding effect. Here, the relationship between exposure and outcome is examined at all levels (categories) of the confounding variable. Finally, the adjusted OR or RR is calculated using a statistical method (Mental Henszel statistics) [2].

Statistical modeling (multivariable analysis, such as logistic regression analysis): This method is most suitable for adjusting for single or multiple confounding factors in a study. All confounding variables are included in a mathematical model to obtain the adjusted values of the measure of association (RR or OR) between exposure and the outcome of interest. This can easily be done using statistical software such as SPSS [7], Stata [8], or others. For more details, readers are referred to the biostatistics book by WW Daniel [9].

15.3.4 Residual Confounding

Incomplete adjustment of confounding effects, or residual confounding, occurs when the confounding effect is not completely removed after adjustment for one or more confounding factors. Residual confounding usually occurs in the following situations [3]:

> *When a confounding factor is too broadly categorized for adjustment:* Imperfect adjustment occurs when a continuous confounding variable is broadly categorized for adjustment. For example, when the number of cigarettes smoked is a confounding factor in the relationship between hypertension and heart disease, and the smoking habit is categorized only as "Yes" or "No" for adjustment. In this situation, there may be inadequate adjustment of the confounding effect due to smoking, leading to residual confounding.

> *Not all important confounding factors are considered for adjustment:* When some of the confounding variables are not included for adjustment in the analysis, residual confounding may occur. For example, there are three confounding factors in a study, but the result is adjusted only for two factors during analysis.

> *When an inappropriate marker of the true confounding variable is used for adjustment:* For example, if social class (measured by income) is a confounding factor in a study and level of education is used as a marker for social class for adjustment.

> *Misclassification of confounding variables:* Misclassification of confounding variables may also result in residual confounding.

15.4 Effect Modification and Interaction

Almost all diseases are of multifactorial etiology. The terms interaction and effect modification are compatible and interchangeably used in epidemiology, though there is a subtle difference between them. Effect modification is defined in terms of the effect of a single exposure on an outcome in different strata (levels) of another variable, whereas interaction is defined in terms of the joint effect of two (or more) exposures on an outcome of interest [10–13]. In other words, in effect modification, the interest is to assess the effect of a single exposure on an outcome at different levels of a third variable, whereas in interaction, the interest is in the joint effect of two (or more) exposures on an outcome. Effect modification can be present with no interaction. Similarly, interaction can also be present without effect modification [10, 11].

15.4.1 Effect Modification

Effect modification is different from confounding. Effect modification is a phenomenon when the strength (magnitude) of association between an exposure and outcome varies according to levels (categories) of a third variable (i.e., the strength of association is modified by the presence of a third factor). The third factor (variable) is called the *effect modifier*. The presence of effect modification can be assessed in stratified analysis, where the association between exposure and outcome is analyzed at each level of the third factor [10, 11].

To understand whether effect modification is present or not (Figure 15.3), the first question is whether there is an association between the exposure of interest and the outcome. If an association is present, is it causal (i.e., the association is not because of confounding or bias)? If it is decided that the association is not because of confounding, calculate the strength of association (OR or RR) between exposure and outcome at each level of the third factor. If the strength of association is the same at different levels of the third factor, effect modification is absent. If the strength of association is different, effect modification is present (i.e., the effect of exposure on outcome is modified by the third factor), and the third factor is the effect modifier in the relationship between the exposure of interest and the outcome.

For example, a researcher is interested in examining the association between hypertension and heart disease (myocardial infarction). He found that there

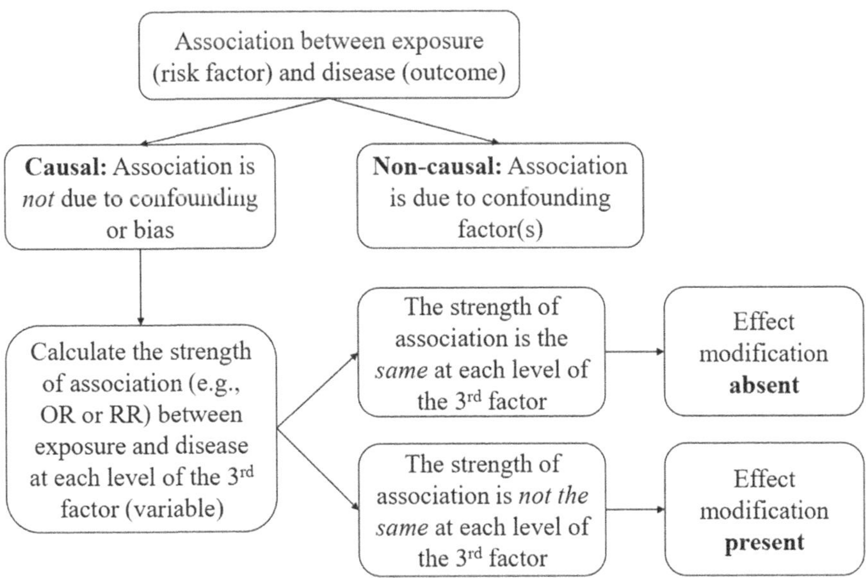

FIGURE 15.3

Schematic diagram to identify effect modification.

Notes: OR: Odds ratio; RR: Relative risk

is a causal association (not confounded by other variables) between hypertension and heart disease. To examine whether the effect of hypertension on heart disease is modified by diabetes, the data were stratified by diabetes (diabetes present/absent), and the strength of association between hypertension and heart disease was checked at each level. If the strength of association (e.g., RR or OR) is similar in two levels of diabetes, effect modification is absent. If it is dissimilar, the relationship between hypertension and heart disease is said to be modified by diabetes (Table 15.4). Here, diabetes is the effect modifier in the relationship between hypertension and heart disease.

Other examples of effect modification are that health education is more effective among the educated group compared to the uneducated, and the risk of coronary heart disease is higher among smokers if there is hypertension, compared to those who do not have hypertension.

A minimum of three factors are required for the phenomenon of effect modification to occur, which include: a) an exposure variable (e.g., hypertension); b) an outcome variable (e.g., heart disease); and c) a potential effect modifier (a third factor such as diabetes or another variable). When effect modification is present, it suggests that two different exposure-disease relationships are operating, one at each level of the third factor. In conclusion, an effect modification is considered to be present if:

- Exposure of interest and disease are causally associated, i.e., the association is not due to one or more confounding factors; and
- When data is stratified by the third variable and if the strength of association between exposure and disease is equally strong across the strata of the third variable, there is no effect modification. If the association is not equally strong across the strata of the third variable, effect modification is present (Figure 15.3 and Table 15.4).

TABLE 15.4

Hypothetical example of the presence or absence of effect modification (Ic: Incidence)

3rd factor: Diabetes	Exposure: Hypertension	Ic. of heart disease per 1,000	Relative Risk (RR)	Effect modification
Present	Absent	5	1.0	Present
	Present	20	4.0	
Absent	Absent	2	1.0	
	Present	4	2.0	
Present	Absent	5	1.0	Absent
	Present	20	4.0	
Absent	Absent	3	1.0	
	Present	12	4.0	

15.4.2 Interaction

Interaction indicates how exposure to multiple risk factors interacts to cause a disease. In interaction, the interest is to assess the effect of two (or more) exposures on the outcome. Interaction may be defined as "when the incidence of a disease in the presence of two or more risk factors differs from the incidence of the disease expected on the basis of their independent effects" [3].

When the incidence of a disease in the presence of two or more risk factors is higher than the expected independent effect, it is called a *positive interaction or synergism*. Conversely, when the incidence of a disease in the presence of two or more risk factors is less than the incidence expected on the basis of their independent effects, it is referred to as *negative interaction or antagonism* [3, 10, 14]. From a clinical and epidemiological point of view, the assessment of interaction in epidemiological studies is important to evaluate the combined effects of two or more drugs in treating a disease or to evaluate the effect of two or more risk factors on an outcome [10].

Interaction between two or more variables may occur in the form of an *additive or multiplicative model* [3, 14]. In the additive model, the effect of interaction is measured by attributable risk (AR), while in the multiplicative model, the effect is measured by relative risk (RR).

15.4.2.1 Additive Interaction Model

In additive interactions, the interaction effect is measured in the form of attributable risk (AR). To explain additive interactions, we have used hypothetical data on incidences of heart disease in the presence or absence of hypertension and diabetes, as shown in Table 15.5 (under "observed incidence rates per 1,000"). The table shows that the incidence of heart disease is five per 1,000 when the study subjects are free from both hypertension and diabetes (cell "a"). This is called the background risk. The cell "b" shows the incidence of heart disease (15 per 1,000) among those who have hypertension alone (without diabetes). Similarly, cell "c" indicates the incidence of heart disease

TABLE 15.5

Additive interaction absent

Observed incidence rates/1,000			Observed attributable risks (AR)/1,000		
	Hypertension			**Hypertension**	
	No	**Yes**		**No**	**Yes**
No diabetes	5.0 (a)	15.0 (b)	No diabetes	0	10.0
Have diabetes	10.0 (c)	20.0 (d)	Have diabetes	5.0	15.0

Expected joint attributable risk (AR) = 10.0 + 5.0 = 15.0
Observed joint AR = 15.0

TABLE 15.6

Additive interaction present

Observed incidence rates/1,000				Observed attributable risks (AR)/1,000		
	Hypertension				Hypertension	
	No	Yes			No	Yes
No diabetes	5.0	15.0	No diabetes		0	10.0
Have diabetes	10.0	30.0	Have diabetes		5.0	25.0

Expected joint attributable risk (AR) = 10.0 + 5.0 = 15.0
Observed joint AR = 25.0

(ten per 1,000) among those who have diabetes alone but not hypertension. When the subjects had both hypertension and diabetes, the incidence was found to be 20 per 1,000 (cell "d"). The next table (under "observed attributable risks per 1,000") shows the attributable risks calculated from the data (measured as incidence among exposed minus incidence among unexposed) (see Section 8.7).

The question is: what is the expected joint attributable risk (AR) if subjects are exposed to both hypertension and diabetes? If the subjects are exposed to both factors, it is expected that the joint effect would be equal to the sum of their individual ARs, i.e., (10.0 + 5.0) or 15.0. Since the expected joint AR is the same as the observed joint AR, there is no interaction (Table 15.5).

However, if the incidence of heart disease were 30 among individuals who have both hypertension and diabetes, the observed joint AR would be 25, which is greater than the expected joint AR of 15 (Table 15.6). This is a situation when we say that there is an additive interaction between hypertension and diabetes in the causation of heart disease.

15.4.2.2 Multiplicative Interaction Model

For the evaluation of multiplicative interactions, the relative risk (RR) is used as the measure of the interaction effect. Let us use the hypothetical data to explain the multiplicative interaction as shown in Table 15.7 (under "observed incidence rates per 1,000"). The data show that the incidence of heart disease among those who have hypertension without diabetes is 15 per 1,000, and that among diabetics without hypertension is ten per 1,000. The joint incidence among individuals exposed to both factors (hypertension and diabetes) is found to be 30 per 1,000. The table under "observed relative risks per 1,000" shows the RRs calculated from the data. The data show that the independent RR of heart disease for hypertension is three, and that of diabetes is two, compared to those who do not have either hypertension or diabetes.

TABLE 15.7

Multiplicative interaction absent

Observed incidence rates/1,000				Observed relative risks (RR)		
	Hypertension				Hypertension	
	No	Yes			No	Yes
No diabetes	5.0	15.0	No diabetes		1.0	3.0
Have diabetes	10.0	30.0	Have diabetes		2.0	6.0

Expected joint relative risk (RR) = 3.0 x 2.0 = 6.0
Observed joint RR = 6.0

TABLE 15.8

Multiplicative interaction present

Observed incidence rates/1,000				Observed relative risks (RR)		
	Hypertension				Hypertension	
	No	Yes			No	Yes
No diabetes	5.0	15.0	No diabetes		1.0	3.0
Have diabetes	10.0	45.0	Have diabetes		2.0	9.0

Expected joint relative risk (RR) = 3.0 x 2.0 = 6.0
Observed joint RR = 9.0

In the multiplicative interaction model, the expected joint effect is the multiplication of the RRs calculated for the exposures independently, which is 6.0 (3.0 x 2.0). Since the expected joint effect and the observed joint effect are the same, there is no interaction (Table 15.7). If the observed joint effect were greater than the expected joint effect, a multiplicative interaction would be present, as shown in Table 15.8. Further clarification of interaction models is provided elsewhere [3, 14].

15.5 How to Identify If Confounding or Effect Modification Is Present

The phenomenon of effect modification and interaction is different from the phenomenon of confounding. Both confounding and effect modification can occur simultaneously for a variable. While the confounding effect can be adjusted for during analysis (Section 15.3.3), it is inappropriate and difficult to adjust for effect modification [3, 15]. It is therefore important to identify if effect modification or confounding is present in the relationship between the exposure of interest and the disease. Notably, when effect modification is present, it can be very difficult to ascertain the presence of confounding. However, to identify whether confounding or effect modification is present, calculate the following three measures of association after stratification of the data by the suspected confounding factor or effect modifier [15].

A: Calculate the crude strength of association (e.g., RR or OR) between the exposure of interest and the disease;

B1: Find the strength of association (e.g., RR or OR) between the exposure of interest and the disease among those who are *exposed* to the potential confounding factor or effect modifier (the third variable). This can be done through stratification of the data by the third factor; and

B2: Determine the strength of association (e.g., RR or OR) between the exposure of interest and the disease among those who are *unexposed* to the potential confounding factor or effect modifier (the third variable).

In general, if the strengths of association between exposure and disease across the strata of the third factor are the same (i.e., B1=B2) but different from the crude association (A), confounding is present, and effect modification is absent. If the strengths of association between exposure and disease at different levels of the third factor are different (i.e., B1 and B2 are different from one another) and at least one of them (B1 or B2) is different from the crude association (A), effect modification is present.

When effect modification is present in a study, calculating an overall measure of association may be inappropriate. Unlike confounding, effect modification is a complex phenomenon that cannot be statistically adjusted for. A common approach to dealing with effect modification is to analyze the data for associations separately at each level (stratum) of the third variable (effect modifier) and to present the strata-specific values [3, 15].

References

1. Delgado-Rodriguez M, Llorca J. Bias. *J Epidemiol Community Health*. 2004;58(8):635–41.
2. Hennekens CH, Buring JE. *Epidemiology in Medicine*. Boston/Toronto: Little Brown and Company; 1987.
3. Szklo M, Nieto FJ. *Epidemiology: Beyond the Basics*. 2nd ed. Boston: Jones and Bartlett Publishers; 2007.
4. Alexander LK, Lopes B, Ricchetti-Masterson K, Yeatts KB. Sources of Systematic Error or Bias: Information Bias. *ERIC Notebook*; 2015;07. Available from:

https://sph.unc.edu/wp-content/uploads/sites/112/2015/07/nciph_ERIC14.pdf.

5. Kumar G, Acharya AS. Biases in epidemiological studies: How far are we from the truth? *Indian J Med Spec.* 2014;5(1):29–35. doi: 10.7713/ijms.2013.0039.

6. Rivas-Ruiz F, Pérez-Vicente S, González-Ramírez AR. Bias in clinical epidemiological study designs. *Allergol Immunopathol (Madr).* 2013;41(1):54–9.

7. Islam MT, Kabir R, Nisha M. *Data Analysis with Stata: A Comprehensive Guide for Data Analysis and Interpretation of Outputs.* Dhaka, Bangladesh: ASA Publications; 2022.

8. Islam MT, Kabir R, Nisha M. *Learning SPSS Without Pain.* 2nd ed. Dhaka, Bangladesh: ASA Publications; 2021.

9. Daniel WW. *Biostatistics: A Foundation for Analysis in the Health Sciences.* 7th ed. New York: John Wiley & Sons; 1999.

10. Corraini P, Olsen M, Pedersen L, Dekkers OM, Vandenbroucke JP. Effect modification, interaction and mediation: An overview of theoretical insights for clinical investigators. *Clin Epidemiol.* 2017;9:331–8.

11. VanderWeele TJ. On the distinction between interaction and effect modification. *Epidemiology.* 2009;20(6):863–71. doi: 10.1097/EDE.0b013e3181ba333c

12. Keele L, Stevenson RT. Causal interaction and effect modification: Same model, different concepts. *Polit Sci Res Methods.* 2021;9(3):641–9. doi: 10.1017/psrm.2020.12

13. Bours MJL. A nontechnical explanation of the counterfactual definition of effect modification and interaction. *J Clin Epidemiol.* 2021;134:113–24.

14. Gordis L. *Epidemiology.* 5th ed. Philadelphia: Elsevier Saunders; 2014.

15. Alexander LK, Lopes B, Ricchetti-Masterson K, Yeatts KB. Confounding Bias: Part II and Effect Measure Modification. *ERIC Notebook*; 2015; 07. Available from: https://sph.unc.edu/wp-content/uploads/sites/112/2015/07/nciph_ERIC12.pdf.

16

Causality in Epidemiology

Mohammad Tajul Islam

In the previous chapters, we discussed the concept of disease causation (Chapter 2), along with the designs and purposes of epidemiological studies. Descriptive studies help us generate hypotheses, which are tested in analytic studies where the presence of an association between exposure and disease is ascertained. The association between exposure and disease refers to the magnitude of the difference between the rates of a disease among the exposed compared to the unexposed group.

One of the primary objectives of epidemiology is to identify the causes of disease. When there is an association between a factor and a disease, it may not suggest that the factor is a cause, especially when there is no logical explanation with the existing knowledge of the biological relationship between the factor and the disease. For instance, if a study finds an association between the presence of TV antennas on rooftops and heart disease, the presence of the antenna cannot be biologically explained as the cause of heart disease.

Identification of causes for a disease is neither simple nor straightforward. It requires judgments based on various factors and evidence. Making judgments about causality from epidemiological data is based on whether the observed association between an exposure and a disease is valid in individual studies and whether the evidence from a number of studies supports the judgment of causality.

When a study finds an association between an exposure and a disease, the observed association may or may not be a true (valid) association. It is important to think about alternative explanations for the association, such as whether the association is due to *chance, bias, or confounding*, before concluding that the association is valid. For causal association, a valid association between an exposure and a disease in a single study is not enough. It is necessary to consider evidence from other studies, biological plausibility, and other factors [1, 2]. This chapter provides a brief overview of alternative

DOI: 10.1201/9781003654803-16

explanations for an association and the guidelines used to assess the presence of a causal relationship.

16.1 Chance or Random Error

Epidemiological studies are conducted by taking a sample from a specified population. When the association between an exposure and a disease is ascertained from a sample, the observed estimate is most likely to be different from the population value (parameter). The observed estimate will also vary from sample to sample if repeated samples are taken from the same population. The difference between the sample value of an estimate and the population value is called the *sampling error or random error*.

A study may find an association between an exposure and a disease even though there is actually no association in the population (a false or spurious association) because of random error or chance. For example, a study might find an association between the use of artificial sweeteners and bladder cancer due to chance or random error, but actually, there is no association in the population. Similarly, because of chance, a study might report a relative risk of 1.3 when the actual relative risk is 1.0 in the population.

Chance can be assessed by using statistical tests, such as the chi-square test or t-test. These tests provide p-values. Conventionally, if the p-value is small (less than 0.05), it is considered that the association is not due to chance. Actually, p-values do not provide any "yes or no" information. A small p-value indicates that it is less likely to find an association between an exposure and a disease by chance. For example, if the p-value of an association is 0.01, it indicates that there is only a 1% probability of obtaining the association when, actually, there is no association in the population (also see Section 17.2.1). It is important to note that a statistical association, when present, does not indicate the existence of a cause-and-effect relationship.

Another way to judge whether the association is by chance or not is to calculate the confidence interval (CI) of the measure (conventionally, the 95% CI). The CI gives a range of values. A narrow range of CI indicates the consistency (less variability) of an estimate. A wide CI indicates higher variability and, thus, a greater possibility of chance. A wide CI also indicates an inadequate sample size in the study.

Random error occurs in all studies. If the sample size is small, there is a greater probability of obtaining an association by chance. Random error cannot be eliminated from a study. However, it can be minimized by taking a large sample (the larger the sample size, the smaller the random error). A large sample reduces the random error.

16.2 Bias and Confounding

Bias is a systematic error resulting from faulty design, selection of study subjects, or procedure of data collection on exposure and/or outcome. Due to bias, the study results can be different from the true results. A study may also find an association between exposure and outcome even though there is no association in the population, in the presence of bias.

Systematic error or bias can be of two types: selection bias and information (or observation) bias. Another type of bias in epidemiological studies is the confounding bias (see Chapter 15). Selection bias occurs because of faulty selection of cases or controls (or exposed or unexposed groups), while information bias occurs due to faulty or inadequate data collection from study subjects, as well as the use of imperfect definitions of variables.

When the strength of association (measured by the odds ratio or relative risk) between an exposure and an outcome of interest is changed due to the presence of a third variable, the phenomenon is called confounding. There can be a false association because of confounding. The presence of confounding can also mask an association between exposure and outcome. The role of chance, bias, and confounding in epidemiological studies is discussed in detail in Chapter 15.

16.3 Hill's Criteria of Causality

Bradford-Hill suggested a set of criteria, which are widely used in epidemiology as a guideline to assess whether an observed association is likely to be causal [3–5]. The following are the viewpoints for the evaluation of a causal relationship as suggested by Hill.

16.3.1 Strength of the Association

In epidemiology, the strength of an association is often measured by relative risk (RR) or odds ratio (OR). The magnitude of the observed association (e.g., RR or OR) is a useful indication of a cause-and-effect relationship. If a factor is strongly associated with a disease, it is more likely that the association is not due to chance or uncontrolled confounding factors. Therefore, the stronger the association between a risk factor and an outcome, the more likely the relationship is causal. However, a small strength of association does not indicate that the association is non-causal.

16.3.2 Temporal Relationship

Temporal relationship is an important evidence to consider for the judgment of causal relationship. It is easier to establish a temporal relationship in prospective cohort studies than in case-control studies. If a factor is said to be the cause of a disease, the exposure must have occurred before the development of the disease by a period of time consistent with a proposed biological mechanism. For example, the latent period for developing lung cancer after exposure to asbestos is 10-15 years. If an individual develops lung cancer after a two-year exposure to asbestos, it may not be the causal factor.

16.3.3 Dose-Response Relationship

The presence of a dose-response relationship is another evidence of causal association. The dose-response relationship indicates that as the dose of exposure increases, the risk of disease also increases. An inverse relationship is also possible, such that the risk of disease decreases as the dose of exposure increases. The presence of a dose-response relationship is strong evidence for a causal association. However, the absence of a dose-response relationship does not necessarily indicate that the association is non-causal.

16.3.4 Consistency of the Association

When similar results are observed in different studies conducted by different investigators using alternative methodologies, in different geographical areas, among diverse populations, and at different times, this supports a causal relationship. For example, the relationship between smoking and coronary heart disease (CHD). Numerous studies have been conducted on the association in different populations over time, using case-control and cohort designs, and consistently found that smoking is associated with an increased risk of CHD [1].

16.3.5 Biological Plausibility

The confidence in causal association is enhanced if there is a known biological mechanism by which exposure causes the disease. For example, consumption of mild to moderate alcohol reduces the risk of CHD. The mechanism by which small or moderate consumption of alcohol reduces the risk of CHD is that alcohol consumption increases high-density lipoprotein (HDL) cholesterol in the blood, which decreases the risk of CHD.

16.3.6 Specificity of the Association

The specificity of association refers to the association when a certain exposure is associated with only one outcome (disease). This is the weakest indication since many exposures are associated with more than one outcome, e.g., cigarette smoking is associated with various cancers, heart disease, and other chronic diseases.

16.3.7 Effect of Cessation of Exposure

If a factor is a cause for a disease, it is expected that the disease incidence will reduce with the reduction or elimination of the factor. Experimental studies can be designed to evaluate the effect of withdrawing a suspected factor on the reduction or prevention of the desired outcome. When the withdrawal of exposure is associated with an alteration in the risk of developing the outcome in experimental studies, it provides evidence of a causal association.

16.3.8 Coherence

This viewpoint has limited utility [5]. To support a causal association, the term coherence implies that any new finding should not be in opposition to the current evidence (i.e., provide evidence against causality). However, it is necessary to evaluate the new finding to ensure that it is not due to bias or confounding before making such a definite conclusion.

16.3.9 Analogy

This is a weak criterion for causality and is dependent on the subjective opinion of a researcher. Analogy means the exposure-outcome relationship is in line with (i.e., analogous to) other established cause-and-effect relationships. An example of an analogy is that while a heart attack may cause chest pain, not all chest pains are due to a heart attack. The absence of analogies does not indicate evidence against causation [4, 6].

In conclusion, Hill's criteria are a set of guidelines used to assess the causal relationship between an exposure and an outcome. An association is more likely to be causal if multiple sources provide different types of evidence.

References

1. Hennekens CH, Buring JE. *Epidemiology in Medicine.* Boston/Toronto: Little, Brown and Company; 1987.
2. Gordis L. *Epidemiology.* 5th ed. Philadelphia: Elsevier Saunders; 2014.
3. Hill AB. The environment and disease: Association or causation? *Proc R Soc Med.* 1965;58(5):295–300.
4. Alexander LK, Lopes B, Ricchetti-Masterson K, et al. *Causality. ERIC Notebook.* 2nd ed. Chapel Hill, NC: UNC Gillings School of Global Public Health; 2015.
5. Shimonovich M, Pearce A, Thomson H, Keyes K, Katikireddi SV. Assessing causality in epidemiology: Revisiting Bradford Hill to incorporate developments in causal thinking. *Eur J Epidemiol.* 2021;36(9):873–87. doi:10.1007/s10654-020-00703-7
6. Weed DL. Analogy in causal inference: Rethinking Austin Bradford Hill's neglected consideration. *Ann Epidemiol.* 2018;28(5):343–6. doi:10.1016/j.annepidem.2018.03.004

17

Sample Size Estimation for Epidemiological Studies

Mohammad Tajul Islam

"How many subjects are needed to conduct a study?" is a fundamental question in epidemiological research. The sample size for a study should be calculated during the planning stage. Taking a larger sample than required to achieve the desired objective results in a waste of resources. On the contrary, a very small sample may lead to significant random error, and the results may not have any practical value. Moreover, when a study is conducted with a small sample size, it is less likely to detect a small difference between two or more estimates. To address the research question, the study should therefore include a sufficient number of subjects.

Statistical methods (formulas) are available to estimate the sample size needed for a study. Depending on the study design and objective, several pieces of information are needed to calculate the sample size. The required information should be obtained from a literature review or personal experience. Sometimes, obtaining this information is challenging.

Statistical methods for calculating the sample size should be considered as a guideline, and factors such as the availability of resources and patients, time limitations, and ethical issues need to be taken into account. This chapter presents the statistical methods of calculating the sample size for the major types of epidemiological studies.

17.1 Sample Size for Cross-Sectional Studies

A common objective in cross-sectional studies is to estimate the prevalence of a disease or a health problem in a population, such as the prevalence (measured as a proportion) of asthma or other diseases. Cross-sectional studies are also conducted to estimate the average (mean) value of an entity in a population, such as the mean birthweight of preterm infants born at less

DOI: 10.1201/9781003654803-17

than 37 weeks of gestational age in a hospital. Therefore, in cross-sectional studies, our interest is either in estimating a proportion or a mean. The formulas for calculating the sample size needed to estimate the population proportion and mean are different and are discussed separately in Sections 17.1.1 and 17.1.2.

17.1.1 Sample Size to Estimate the Population Proportion

To calculate the sample size for a cross-sectional study estimating the population proportion, the following formula (Formula 17.1) is used when sampling from an infinite population [1–3]. This formula can also be used when the sampled population is large enough to avoid a finite population correction. A finite population correction is unnecessary if the sample size is ≤5% of the population size.

$$n = \frac{Z^2_{(1-\alpha/2)}PQ}{d^2} \qquad\qquad \left[\text{Formula 17.1}\right]$$

Where

- n is the desired sample size;
- Z is the value from the standard normal distribution at a specified level of significance (α);
- P is the anticipated population proportion;
- Q is (1 – P);
- d is the allowable error (absolute precision required on either side of the estimated proportion); and
- Alpha (α) is the level of significance.

If sampling is planned from a finite population or when a finite population correction is needed, the following formula (Formula 17.2) is used to calculate the sample size:

$$n = \frac{NZ^2_{(1-\alpha/2)}PQ}{d^2(N-1)+Z^2_{(1-\alpha/2)}PQ} \qquad\qquad \left[\text{Formula 17.2}\right]$$

Where N is the study population size and others are the same as above.

The finite population correction can also be done using the following formula (Formula 17.3) after calculating the sample size with the infinite population formula (Formula 17.1):

$$\text{Corrected sample size, } n_c = \frac{n}{1 + \dfrac{n}{N}} \qquad \left[\text{Formula 17.3}\right]$$

Where

- n is the uncorrected sample size calculated using Formula 17.1; and
- N is the study population size.

Example
A researcher plans to conduct a study to estimate the prevalence of asthma among the adult population (aged 20 or older) in a district. The prevalence of asthma in the study population is anticipated to be around 15%. How many subjects should be included in the study to estimate the prevalence of asthma with a 95% confidence level (or 5% level of significance) and a 3% margin of error? Suppose that the total adult population (age greater than 20) in the district is 200,000.

Note that if the sample size is calculated using a 3% error, the 95% confidence interval for the prevalence will fall within the range of "calculated prevalence (%) ± 3%."

From the question above, we have the following information:

- $P = 15\%$ or 0.15;
- $Q = (1 - P)$ or 0.85;
- $\alpha = 0.05$;
- $Z_{(1 - \alpha/2)} = 1.96$ (it is the value of Z when α is 5%) (Table 17.2); and
- $d = 3\%$ or 0.03.

Using Formula 17.1, the calculated sample size is 544.2. It is necessary to round up the calculated sample size to the next whole number. Therefore, the required sample size for the study is 545.

In this example, the calculated sample size is about 0.27% of the study population (545 out of 200,000) in the district. It is therefore not necessary to adjust the sample size for a finite population (since the sample size is less than 5% of the population size). However, if the sample size is adjusted for a finite population (using Formula 17.3), the corrected sample size would be 544, which is essentially the same as the uncorrected sample size.

Let me give an example of when a finite population correction is useful. Suppose that a researcher intends to estimate the proportion of skilled birth attendants (SBAs) who conduct home deliveries in a district. It is anticipated that about 30% of SBAs conduct home deliveries. The researcher wants to calculate the sample size with a 5% level of significance and a 5% margin of error. Information collected from the district health office indicates that there are only 170 SBAs (N) in the district.

Using the above information and Formula 17.1, the calculated sample size is 323, which is greater than the target population size (N=170). In this situation, we have two options: a) study the entire population (N=170) if possible; or b) use the finite population correction (using Formula 17.3 or calculating the sample size using Formula 17.2), which will reduce the required sample size. As mentioned earlier, a finite population correction is recommended when the calculated sample size exceeds 5% of the population size. If we apply the finite population correction using Formula 17.3, the required sample size for the study would be 112.

Other issues that need to be considered when calculating the sample size include adjustments for the design effect and non-response. When cluster sampling is planned for selecting study subjects, the sample size must be adjusted for the design effect, as cluster sampling reduces the effective sample size. The design effect is the ratio of the variance when cluster sampling is used to the variance when simple random sampling is used. The design effect can vary across variables. It is desirable to find an estimated design effect from similar studies through a literature review before calculating the sample size. If such a value is found, it should be used to adjust the sample size.

In reality, most studies do not report the design effect. However, in health-related studies where information about the design effect is unavailable, it is common practice to assume a design effect between 1.5 and 2.0. To adjust the sample size for the design effect, multiply the calculated sample size by the estimated design effect. For example, if the calculated sample size is 545 and the estimated design effect is 2.0, the adjusted sample size would be 1,090 (545 × 2).

To adjust for nonresponse, divide the calculated sample size by "(1 − the proportion of nonresponse)". For example, if a 10% nonresponse rate is anticipated, the final sample size would be 1,212 (1,090 ÷ 0.9).

Occasionally, obtaining an appropriate value for P (anticipated prevalence) may be difficult. When no information is available to estimate P, it is common practice to use a value of P at 50% (0.50). A P value of 0.50 will yield the largest sample size for a fixed value of d (allowable error). However, it is important to be realistic when considering P as 0.5. When different values of P are available in the literature, use the P value that is closest to 50%. For example, if one study indicates a prevalence of 30% and another indicates 40%, use 40% as the P value to calculate the sample size. Similarly, if the proportion is assumed to be between 60% and 70%, use 60% for the sample size calculation [4].

Another important issue is deciding the appropriate value for d, also known as the allowable error or margin of error. There are no definitive guidelines for selecting the value for d. Researchers commonly use 5% (0.05) as the value for d, regardless of the value of P (anticipated prevalence). One publication suggests using 5% (0.05) for d if the anticipated prevalence is between 20% and 80% [4], while another report recommends using 5% for d if the anticipated prevalence is between 10% and 90% [5].

However, if the anticipated prevalence is less than 20% or greater than 80%, the value of d should be considered relative to the anticipated prevalence (relative precision). For instance, if the prevalence of a condition in the population is anticipated to be 10%, a relative precision of 20% (or 15%) may be considered for d. In this case, the value of d would be 2% or 0.02 (20% of 10) for the sample size calculation.

17.1.2 Sample Size to Estimate the Population Mean

In cross-sectional studies, where the objective is to estimate the population mean, the following formula should be used when the population is infinite or when finite population correction is not required [1–3]:

$$n = \frac{Z^2_{(1-\alpha/2)}\sigma^2}{d^2} \qquad \left[\text{Formula } 17.4\right]$$

Where

- n is the desired sample size;
- Z is the value from the standard normal distribution at a specified level of significance (α);
- σ is the anticipated standard deviation of the estimate;
- d is the allowable error or desired margin of error (absolute precision required on either side of the mean); and
- Alpha (α) is the level of significance.

For a finite population or when a finite population correction is needed, the formula to calculate the sample size is:

$$n = \frac{NZ^2_{(1-\alpha/2)}\sigma^2}{d^2(N-1)+Z^2_{(1-\alpha/2)}\sigma^2} \qquad \left[\text{Formula } 17.5\right]$$

Where N is the study population size, and others are the same as above.

The finite population correction can also be done using Formula 17.3 after calculating the sample size with Formula 17.4.

Example

An investigator wants to estimate the mean birthweight of infants born to mothers who had hypertension during pregnancy. The investigator plans to collect data from birth records at a hospital. Previous studies indicate that the standard deviation of birthweights of infants born in hospitals ranges from 650 g to 670 g. If the researcher aims to estimate the sample size with a 5% level of significance and a margin of error of 100 g, what would be the required sample size for the study? Note that if the sample size is calculated using a margin of error of 100 g, the 95% confidence interval (CI) for the estimated mean will lie within the range of "mean ± 100 g."

From the above example, we have:

- $Z_{(1-\alpha/2)} = 1.96$ (it is the value of Z when α is 5%);
- $\alpha = 0.05$;
- $\sigma = 650$ g to 670 g (we will consider the higher value to get a larger sample); and
- $d = 100$ g.

For an infinite population, the sample size can be calculated by using Formula 17.4, and the required sample size for the study would be 173.

If 5% of the hospital records lack birthweight information, the sample size after adjusting for missing data will be 183 [173 ÷ (1 − 0.05)]. Therefore, the investigator is required to review 183 birth records to obtain 173 complete data.

In hospital-based studies, cluster sampling methods are usually unnecessary for selecting the study subjects. However, for a community-based study where cluster sampling is planned, the sample size requires adjustment for the design effect, as discussed in Section 17.1.1.

17.2 Sample Size for Hypothesis Testing

17.2.1 Type I and Type II Errors

The majority of studies are conducted by taking a sample from the population to test a hypothesis. Suppose that a researcher conducted a study to determine whether there is an association between obesity and diabetes by taking a sample from a specified population. In this case, the null hypothesis (H_0) is "there is no association between obesity and diabetes," while the alternative hypothesis is "there is an association between obesity and diabetes".

To test the hypothesis, if the researcher uses the chi-square test, the test result will either reject or not reject the null hypothesis at a specific level of significance (e.g., at a 5% level of significance). The study results, in relation to the actual association in the population, will lead to one of four possible outcomes, as shown in Table 17.1.

TABLE 17.1

Results of a hypothesis test in relation to the actual situation in the population

		In the population	
		Association (H_0 rejected)	**No association** (H_0 not rejected)
Study result says	Association (H_0 rejected)	[a] Correct conclusion	[b] Type I error (α)
	No association (H_0 not rejected)	[c] Type II error (β)	[d] Correct conclusion

The study result may indicate an association (if the null hypothesis is rejected) when there is also an association in the population (cell a). Similarly, the study result may indicate no association when there is also no association in the population (cell d). These represent correct conclusions (cells a and d). However, since the true state of association in the population is unknown, we cannot confirm these conclusions. We need to consider the following alternatives.

First, it may happen that the study result shows an association, but in fact, there is no association in the population (cell "b"). Drawing a conclusion based on these study findings would result in an incorrect decision (error). The probability of making such a conclusion is called the Type I error (denoted by α). *Therefore, a Type I error represents the probability of rejecting the null hypothesis when there is no association in the population.* This error is indicated by the p-value of the statistical test used for hypothesis testing. For example, if the p-value of the chi-square test for the association between obesity and diabetes is 0.02 (leading to the rejection of the null hypothesis at the 5% level of significance), the Type I error is 0.02 (2%). This indicates a 2% chance (probability) that there is no association in the population, even though the study result suggests an association. A Type I error is sometimes called a "false positive" association.

Second, another situation is that the study result shows no association, but in fact, an association exists in the population (cell "c"). Drawing a conclusion based on these study findings would also lead to an incorrect decision. The probability of making such a conclusion is called the Type II error (denoted by β). *Therefore, a Type II error is the probability of not rejecting the null hypothesis when there is an association in the population.* Type II error is usually not reported in study results but can be calculated using statistical methods. It is often called a "false negative" association. The quantity $(1 - \beta)$ is known as the power of the study.

When planning a study for hypothesis testing, the sample size needs to be sufficiently large to minimize the Type I and Type II errors, as discussed above.

17.2.2 Hypothesis Testing: Sample Size for the Difference Between Two Proportions

The sample size needed to test the hypothesis that two independent population proportions are equal can be calculated using Formula 17.6 [2, 3]. To determine the sample size, the following information is needed:

a) The estimated population proportion in the comparison area (P_0);

b) The anticipated population proportion in the intervention (other) area (P_1);

c) The estimated effect size $(P_0 - P_1)$;

d) The level of significance (α); and

e) The power of the study $(1 - \beta)$.

Example

A health intervention program aims to increase the institutional (hospital) delivery rate. To evaluate the impact of the intervention on improving hospital delivery rate, two comparable districts have been selected: one for the intervention (intervention district) and the other for comparison (without intervention). The baseline hospital delivery rate is estimated at 40% in both districts. If the intervention is expected to increase the hospital delivery rate by at least 20%, what sample size (number of women with recent deliveries) would be required for the study, considering a 5% level of significance and 80% power?

The following formula can be used to estimate the sample size for a two-sided test:

$$n = \frac{[Z_{\alpha/2}\sqrt{2PQ} + Z_\beta\sqrt{(P_1 Q_1 + P_0 Q_0)}]^2}{(P_1 - P_0)^2} \qquad \left[\text{Formula 17.6}\right]$$

Where

- n is the desired sample size for each district;

- Z is the value from the standard normal distribution at a specified level of significance (α) and power $(1 - \beta)$;

- Alpha (α) is the level of significance;

- Beta (β) is the type II error, while $(1 - \beta)$ is the power of the study;

- P_0 is the estimated proportion of outcome (hospital delivery rate) in the comparison district (or unexposed group);

- Q_0 is $(1 - P_0)$;

- P_1 is the estimated proportion of the outcome in the intervention district (exposed group) after the intervention;

- Q_1 is $(1 - P_1)$;

- $P = \dfrac{\left(P_1 + P_0\right)}{2}$; and

- Q is $(1 - P)$.

The quantities $Z_{\alpha/2}$ and Z_β are values derived from the standard normal distribution (Z-distribution) table corresponding to the values of α and β. Table 17.2 shows the values of Z_α and Z_β for the commonly used values of α and β. From the above problem, we have:

- Level of significance (α) is 5%;
- Power of the study $(1 - \beta)$ is 80% (i.e., β is 0.20);
- $Z_{\alpha/2}$ is 1.96 (Table 17.2);
- Z_β is 0.84 (Table 17.2);
- P_0 is 40.0% or 0.40;
- Q_0 is $(1 - P_0)$ or 0.60;
- P_1 is 48.0% or 0.48 [if there is an increase of 20% from the baseline (40%), the expected hospital delivery rate is 48%];
- Q_1 is 0.52;
- P is 0.44; and
- Q is 0.56.

Therefore, the sample size required for the study is 592 women for each district (total sample size is 1,184). Note that if cluster sampling is used for data

TABLE 17.2

Values of Z_α and Z_β for selected values of α and β

α or β	One-sided test Z_α and Z_β	Two-sided test $Z_{\alpha/2}$
0.001	3.09	3.29
0.005	2.58	2.81
0.01	2.33	2.58
0.025	1.96	2.24
0.05	1.64	1.96
0.10	1.28	1.64
0.20	0.84	1.28
0.30	0.52	1.04

Note: The values of Z_β are the same for both one-sided and two-sided tests of significance and therefore, consider the value under one-sided test.

collection, the sample size needs to be adjusted for the design effect (Section 17.1.1). Similarly, adjustments for non-response should also be considered.

Alternatively, Formula 17.7 can be used to calculate the sample size for testing the hypothesis for a difference between two population proportions [2]. This formula will yield a sample size equivalent to the earlier method. The formula is:

$$\text{Sample size, } n = 2 \times \frac{(Z_{\alpha/2} + Z_{\beta})^2}{ES^2} \qquad \left[\text{Formula } 17.7\right]$$

$$\text{Effect size, } ES = \frac{|P_1 - P_2|}{\sqrt{P(1-P)}}$$

Where

- n is the desired sample size for each district;
- Z is the value from the standard normal distribution at a specified level of significance (α) and power ($1 - \beta$);
- Alpha (α) is the level of significance;
- Beta (β) is the type II error, while ($1 - \beta$) is the power of the study;
- ES is the effect size;
- P_1 is the estimated proportion of outcome (hospital delivery rate) in the comparison district (or unexposed group);
- P_2 is the estimated proportion of outcome in the intervention district (or exposed group) after the intervention;
- $P = \dfrac{(P_1 + P_2)}{2}$; and
- $|P_1 - P_2|$ indicates absolute difference between P_1 and P_2.

17.2.3 Hypothesis Testing: Sample Size for the Difference Between Two Proportions Before and After Intervention in a Single Population

The sample size required to determine the difference between two population proportions can be calculated for a study with a pre-test and post-test evaluation (before and after intervention) conducted within a single population. The sample size for such a study design can be calculated using the following formula [3]:

$$n = \frac{[Z_{\alpha/2}\sqrt{P_0 Q_0} + Z_{\beta}\sqrt{P_1 Q_1}]^2}{(P_0 - P_1)^2} \qquad \left[\text{Formula } 17.8\right]$$

Where

- n is the desired sample size;
- Z is the value from the standard normal distribution at a specified level of significance (α) and power ($1 - \beta$);
- Alpha (α) is the level of significance;
- Beta (β) is the type II error, while ($1 - \beta$) is the power of the study;
- P_0 is the baseline (before intervention) prevalence of the outcome of interest (e.g., a disease);
- Q_0 is ($1 - P_0$);
- P_1 is the anticipated prevalence after intervention; and
- Q_1 is ($1 - P_1$).

Example
An investigator plans an intervention program with the aim of reducing the prevalence of sexually transmitted infections (STIs) among female commercial sex workers (CSWs) in a brothel. To evaluate the impact, the investigator decided to use a pre- and post-intervention design. A recent study shows that the prevalence of STIs among female CSWs is 15%. How many female CSWs are required to enroll in this study if it is anticipated that the intervention will reduce the prevalence of STIs by at least five percentage points (a 33% reduction), with a 95% confidence level and 80% power?
From the example above, we have the following information:

- Level of significance (α) is 5%;
- Power of the study ($1 - \beta$) is 80% or β is 0.20;
- $Z_{\alpha/2}$ is 1.96 (Table 17.2);
- Z_β is 0.84 (Table 17.2);
- P_0 is 15% or 0.15;
- Q_0 is ($1 - 0.15$) or 0.85;
- P_1 is 10% or 0.10; and
- Q_1 is ($1 - 0.10$) or 0.90.

Using Formula 17.8, the minimum sample size required for the study is 363 female CSWs before the intervention and 363 after the intervention.

17.2.4 Hypothesis Testing: Sample Size for the Difference Between Two Independent Population Means

In studies where the objective is to test a hypothesis to compare the means of a continuous outcome between two independent populations, the following formula (Formula 17.9) is used to calculate the required sample size:

$$\text{Sample size, n} = 2 \times \frac{\left(Z_{\alpha/2} + Z_{\beta}\right)^2}{ES^2} \qquad \left[\text{Formula 17.9}\right]$$

$$\text{Effect size, ES} = \frac{|\mu_1 - \mu_2|}{\sigma}$$

Where

- n is the required sample size in each group;
- Z is the value from the standard normal distribution for the specified values of α (level of significance) and β (Type II error);
- Alpha (α) is the level of significance;
- Beta (β) is the Type II error, while $(1 - \beta)$ is the power of the study;
- μ_1 is the estimated population mean of the outcome variable in one group;
- μ_2 is the estimated population mean of the outcome variable in the other group;
- $|\mu_1 - \mu_2|$ indicates absolute difference between μ_1 and μ_2;
- σ is the standard deviation of the outcome variable; and
- ES is the effect size.

Example

An investigator aims to compare the mean birthweight of infants born to mothers with and without hypertension during pregnancy. Previous studies report that the mean birthweight of infants born to women without pregnancy complications is 2,900 g, with a standard deviation of 550 g. The anticipated mean birthweight of infants born to hypertensive women is 2,700 g. How many newborns are required to detect this difference at a 5% level of significance and 80% power?

From the above example, we have the following information:

- Level of significance (α) is 5%, so that $Z_{\alpha/2}$ is 1.96 (Table 17.2);
- Power $(1 - \beta)$ of the study is 80%, so that Z_{β} is 0.84 (Table 17.2);
- μ_1 is 2,900 g;

- μ_2 is 2,700 g; and
- σ is 550 g.

The required sample size for this study is 119 in each group, i.e., 119 newborns born to mothers with hypertension and 119 newborns born to mothers without hypertension.

For the calculation of sample size when the standard deviations (SDs) of both groups are available in the literature, it is preferable to calculate the pooled SD (see references [1, 2] for the formula) and use it to estimate the sample size. However, commonly, the SD of the unexposed group (women without hypertension) is available, and the value can be used to calculate the sample size.

17.2.5 Hypothesis Testing: Sample Size for the Difference Between Two Related Sample Means

When the objective of a study is to compare the means of two related samples (e.g., in a matched pairs or a before-after design), the following formula can be used to calculate the sample size.

$$\text{Sample size, n} = \frac{(Z_{\alpha/2} + Z_\beta)^2}{ES^2} \qquad \left[\text{Formula 17.10}\right]$$

$$\text{Effect size, ES} = \frac{|\mu_2 - \mu_1|}{\sigma_d}$$

Where

- n is the required sample size in each group;
- Z is the value from the standard normal distribution for the specified values of α (level of significance) and β (Type II error);
- Alpha (α) is the level of significance;
- Beta (β) is the Type II error, while $(1 - \beta)$ is the power of the study;
- μ_1 is the estimated mean of the outcome variable in one group (or before intervention);
- μ_2 is the estimated mean of the outcome variable in the other group (or after intervention);
- ES is the effect size;
- $|\mu_1 - \mu_2|$ indicates absolute difference between μ_1 and μ_2; and
- σ_d is the standard deviation of the difference in outcome variable.

Example

A researcher plans to conduct a study to determine if nutritional counseling (intervention) during pregnancy increases blood hemoglobin levels. To conduct the study, the researcher plans to enroll a group of pregnant women and measure their hemoglobin levels before and after receiving nutritional counseling. Previous studies report that the mean hemoglobin level of pregnant women is 9.0 gm%. It is expected that the intervention will increase the mean hemoglobin level by at least 2 gm%. If the standard deviation of the difference in hemoglobin levels before and after the intervention is 4 gm%, how many pregnant women are needed for the study to test the hypothesis at a 5% level of significance and 90% power?

From the example, we have the following information:

- Level of significance (α) is 5%, so that $Z_{\alpha/2}$ is 1.96 (Table 17.2);
- Power ($1 - \beta$) of the study is 90%, so that Z_{β} is 1.28 (Table 17.2);
- μ_1 is 9.0 gm%;
- μ_2 is 11.0 gm%; and
- σ_d is 4.0 gm%.

The required sample size for this study is 42 pregnant women, before and after the intervention.

17.3 Sample Size for Case-Control Studies

Case-control studies are generally conducted to identify risk factors for a disease. In case-control studies, the strength of the association is measured by the odds ratio (OR). Primarily, there are two types of case-control studies: unmatched and matched case-control studies. The number of subjects required for a case-control study depends on the specification of the following four factors:

1) Proportion of controls exposed to the risk factor of interest (i.e., the prevalence of exposure among the control group) in the target population (P_0);

2) Anticipated minimum odds ratio (or relative risk) associated with the exposure of interest that would have sufficient public health importance (R);

3) Desired level of significance (α); and

4) Desired power of the study ($1 - \beta$).

17.3.1 Sample Size for an Unmatched Case-Control Study

In unmatched case-control studies, controls are not matched with cases on any characteristics. In such designs, the case-to-control ratio can vary from 1:1 to 1:4. Therefore, the formula for the calculation of sample size in an unmatched design depends on the ratio of cases to controls [6].

17.3.1.1 Sample Size for Equal Number of Cases and Controls

If an equal number of cases and controls (a case-control ratio of 1:1) is considered for the study, the required sample size in each group is calculated using the following formula:

$$\text{Sample size, n} = \frac{2pq(Z_{\alpha/2} + Z_{\beta})^2}{(P_1 - P_0)^2} \qquad [\text{Formula } 17.11]$$

Where

- $P_1 = \dfrac{P_0 R}{1 + P_0(R-1)};$

- $p = \dfrac{(P_1 + P_0)}{2};$

- $q = (1-p);$

- $q = (1-p);$

- P_0 is the proportion of controls exposed to the risk factor of interest;

- R is the anticipated minimum odds ratio (or relative risk) associated with the exposure of interest;

- α is the desired level of significance;

- β is the Type II error, while $(1 - \beta)$ is the power of the study; and

- $Z_{\alpha/2}$ and Z_{β} are values from the standard normal distribution (Z-distribution) corresponding to the values of α (two-sided) and β.

Example

Suppose a researcher aims to determine whether undernutrition is a risk factor for persistent diarrhea (diarrhea lasting more than 14 days) among children under five years of age. To test the hypothesis, the researcher designed a hospital-based unmatched case-control study with a 1:1 case-to-control ratio. The cases for this study are children with persistent diarrhea, while the controls are children with diarrhea lasting less than 14 days. How many cases and controls are needed to conduct the study if the goal is to detect a minimum odds ratio of 2.0, with a 5% level of significance and 80% power?

From the problem above, we have the following information for the calculation of sample size:

- Anticipated minimum odds ratio to be detected in the study, R (= 2.0);
- The level of significance, $\alpha = 0.05$ ($Z_{\alpha/2} = 1.96$, obtained from Table 17.2 for a two-sided test); and
- Power of the study $(1 - \beta)$ is 80% ($Z_\beta = 0.84$, obtained from Table 17.2).

The above problem did not provide any information on the prevalence of undernutrition in the control group, which is required for sample size calculation. Previous studies suggest the prevalence of undernutrition among under-5 children suffering from acute diarrhea is 20.0% (i.e., $P_0 = 0.20$). If data on the prevalence of undernutrition among children with acute diarrhea is not available, the prevalence of undernutrition among under-5 children in the general population can be considered instead. Therefore,

- $P_1 = \dfrac{0.2 \times 2}{1 + 0.2(2 - 1)} = 0.33;$

- $p = 0.27;$ and

- $q = 0.73.$

The required sample size for the study is 175 in each group, i.e., the study requires 175 cases and 175 controls.

17.3.1.2 Sample Size for Multiple Controls per Case

A simple extension of Formula 17.11 gives an estimation of sample size with multiple controls per case. With "C" controls per case, the formula for calculating the sample size is given below (Formula 17.12). Here, "n" indicates the number of cases, while "(C x n)" is the number of controls required for the study.

$$\text{Sample size, n} = \frac{pq(1 + 1/C)(Z_{\alpha/2} + Z_\beta)^2}{(P_1 - P_0)^2} \qquad [\text{Formula } 17.12]$$

Where

- $P_1 = \dfrac{P_0 R}{1 + P_0(R - 1)};$

- $p = \dfrac{(P_1 + P_0)}{2}$;

- $q = (1 - p)$;

- C is the number of controls per case;

- P_0 is the proportion of controls exposed to the risk factor of interest;

- R is the anticipated minimum odds ratio (or relative risk) associated with the exposure of interest;

- α is the desired level of significance;

- β is the Type II error, while (1 – β) is the power of the study; and

- $Z_{\alpha/2}$ and Z_{β} are the values from the standard normal distribution (Z-distribution) corresponding to specific the values of α (two sided) and β.

If we consider the above example of an unmatched case-control study and decide to take two controls per case, the required sample size for the study is 130 cases and 260 controls.

17.3.2 Sample Size for a Matched Case-Control Design

In matched case-control studies, data are presented in pairs. As discussed in Section 7.8.3, matched case-control data are analyzed based on discordant pairs. The sample size for a matched case-control study can be calculated using the following formulas (Formulas 17.13 and 17.14):

$$\text{No. of discordant pairs, } m = \frac{[Z_{\alpha/2}/2 + Z_{\beta}\sqrt{P(1-P)}]^2}{(P-0.5)^2} \qquad [\text{Formula } 17.13]$$

Where

- $P = R/(1+R)$;

- R represents the estimated minimum odds ratio to be detected in the study; and

- $Z_{\alpha/2}$ and Z_{β} are values from the standard normal distribution (Z-distribution) corresponding to the values of α (two-sided) and β.

The following formula gives the sample size (number of pairs) required for the study:

Sample size (no. of pairs), $M = \dfrac{m}{\left(p_0 q_1 + p_1 q_0\right)}$ [Formula 17.14]

Where

- $p_1 = \dfrac{p_0 R}{1 + p_0 (R-1)}$;

- p_0 is the estimated prevalence of exposure among controls in the target population;

- R is the estimated (minimum) odds ratio to be detected in the study;

- $q_0 = (1 - p_0)$; and

- $q_1 = (1 - p_1)$.

Example

Suppose a researcher plans to determine whether undernutrition is a risk factor for persistent diarrhea (diarrhea lasting more than 14 days) among children under five years of age. To test the hypothesis, the researcher has designed a hospital-based matched case-control study (matched for gender). The cases for this study are children with persistent diarrhea, while the controls are children with diarrhea for less than 14 days. It is known from a previous study that the prevalence of undernutrition among children with acute diarrhea is 20%. How many pairs of cases and controls does the study need if it is intended to detect a minimum odds ratio of 2.0 at a 5% level of significance and 80% power?

From the problem above, we have the following information:

- The minimum odds ratio to be detected in the study, R (= 2.0);
- Prevalence of exposure (undernutrition) among the control group (p_0) is 20%;
- The level of significance, $\alpha = 0.05$ ($Z_{\alpha/2} = 1.96$, obtained from Table 17.2 for a two-sided test); and
- Power of the study $(1 - \beta)$ is 80% ($Z_\beta = 0.84$, obtained from Table 17.2).

With the above information, we can calculate the values for:

- P (= 0.67);
- p_1 (= 0.33);
- q_0 (= 0.8); and
- q_1 (= 0.67).

Using Formulas 17.13 and 17.14, the total number of case-control pairs required for this study is 165 (i.e., 165 cases and 165 controls matched for gender).

17.4 Sample Size for Cohort Studies

In cohort studies, exposed and unexposed groups are followed for a specified period of time to observe the occurrence of an outcome of interest. The strength of the association between exposure and outcome is measured by the relative risk (RR). The following formula can be used to calculate the sample size for a cohort study [3, 7]:

$$n = \frac{[Z_{\alpha/2}\sqrt{2PQ} + Z_{\beta}\sqrt{P_1 Q_1 + P_2 Q_2}]^2}{(P_1 - P_2)^2} \qquad [\text{Formula } 17.15]$$

Where

- n is the required sample size in each group (exposed and unexposed);
- $Z_{\alpha/2}$ and Z_{β} are values from the standard normal distribution (Z-distribution) corresponding to the specific values of α (two-sided) and β;
- α is the desired level of significance;
- β is the Type II error, while $(1 - \beta)$ is the power of the study;
- P_1 is the probability (incidence) of an outcome (e.g., a disease) in the unexposed group;
- P_2 is the probability (incidence) of the outcome in the exposed group;
- $P = \dfrac{P_1 + P_2}{2}$;
- $Q = (1 - P)$;
- $Q_1 = (1 - P_1)$; and
- $Q_2 = (1 - P_2)$.

Example
Suppose that an investigator aims to estimate the risk of death among COVID-19 patients associated with diabetes mellitus in a cohort study. To conduct the study, the investigator plans to include a group of COVID-19 patients with diabetes (exposed) and another group without diabetes (unexposed)

and follow them for a period of six months. The incidence of death among COVID-19 patients without any comorbidity is estimated as 3% in a recent study. How many COVID-19 patients does the researcher need to enroll in the study if it is anticipated that the incidence of death in the exposed group will be 7.5% at a 5% level of significance and 90% power?

From the example above, we have the following information:

- The level of significance, α = 0.05 ($Z_{\alpha/2}$ = 1.96, obtained from Table 17.2 for a two-sided test);
- Power (1 – β) of the study is 90% (Z_{β} = 1.28, obtained from Table 17.2);
- Incidence of death in the unexposed (without any comorbidity) group, P_1 (= 3% or 0.03);
- Anticipated incidence of death among the exposed group (P_2) (= 7.5% or 0.075);
- P is 5.25% or 0.0525;
- Q is 0.9475;
- Q_1 is 0.97; and
- Q_2 is 0.925.

The sample size for the study is 514 in each group, i.e., the study needs 514 COVID-19 patients with diabetes (exposed) and 514 COVID-19 patients without comorbidities (unexposed). If the incidence of death in the exposed and unexposed groups is considered at 3.0% and 2.0%, respectively, the required sample size (to detect a one percent difference) will increase significantly. In this case, the sample size needed will be 5,115 in each group.

An alternative formula for calculating the sample size for cohort studies is also available (Formula 17.16). This formula is based on the relative risk (RR) of exposure that the researcher wants to estimate from the cohort study.

$$n = \frac{[Z_{\alpha/2}\sqrt{2PQ} + Z_{\beta}\sqrt{P_1\{1 + RR - P_1(1 + RR)^2\}}]^2}{P_1^2(RR - 1)} \qquad [\text{Formula } 17.16]$$

Where

- n is the required sample size in each group (exposed and unexposed);
- $Z_{\alpha/2}$ and Z_{β} are values from the standard normal distribution (Z-distribution) corresponding to the specified values of α (two-sided) and β;
- α is the desired level of significance;
- β is the Type II error, while (1 – β) is the power of the study;
- RR is the estimated minimum relative risk of public health importance;

- P_1 is the probability (incidence) of an outcome (e.g., a disease) in the unexposed group;

- $P = \dfrac{P_1(1+RR)}{2}$; and

- $Q = (1-P)$.

The sample size can also be calculated for estimating the incidence of a disease (or a health-related condition) in a single population using the following formula [3]:

$$\text{Sample size, n} = (Z_{\alpha/2} \div d)^2 \qquad [\text{Formula 17.17}]$$

Where d is the relative precision and $Z_{\alpha/2}$ is the value from the standard normal distribution (Z-distribution) corresponding to the specified value of α (two-sided).

Suppose a researcher aims to determine the incidence of pre-eclampsia among pregnant women aged more than 30 years. If the researcher intends to detect the incidence with a 5% relative precision, the estimated minimum sample size required for the study is 1,537, as shown below.

$$\text{Sample size, n} = (1.96 \div 0.05)^2 = 1,537$$

17.5 Sample Size for Clinical Trials

While planning a clinical trial, researchers need to answer some key questions. For instance, a researcher plans to conduct a double-blind randomized controlled trial to compare the effectiveness of drug A against drug B in reducing deaths among patients after an acute heart attack (myocardial infarction, or MI). Before calculating the sample size, the researcher needs to answer the following key questions [8]:

- *What is the main purpose of the study?* Considering the example above, the main purpose of the study is to determine if drug A is more effective in reducing deaths after MI compared to drug B.

- *What is the principal measure of patient outcome?* Death from any cause within one year of follow-up after treatment is considered the outcome of interest.

- *How will the data be analyzed to determine the treatment difference, and at what level of significance?* To detect the significance of the difference in deaths between drug A and drug B, a chi-square test will be applied at a 5% level of significance. Life table analysis can be used to determine survival probability, but calculating the sample size based on life table analysis would be more difficult.

- *What type of results does one anticipate with the standard treatment?* Drug B is considered the standard treatment for MI, and previous studies estimated that approximately 10% of patients die within one year of an acute attack of MI.

- *How small a treatment difference is important to detect, and with what degree of certainty (power of the study)?* To detect a large treatment difference, a smaller sample size is required. However, it is important to consider the detection of a smaller (minimum) difference, which is of clinical importance. The researcher also needs to decide on the power of the study, usually between 80% and 90%.

Given the information above, one can calculate the sample size for a clinical trial. The formula to be used to calculate the sample size depends on the type of outcome measure and the statistic to be used to analyze the data. In clinical trials, usually the outcome measure is either a proportion (for a dichotomous categorical variable) or a mean (for a continuous variable).

17.5.1 Sample Size When the Outcome Measure Is a Proportion (Qualitative Outcome)

When a dichotomous qualitative outcome is considered, the treatment outcome of patients can be categorized as either "success" (indicating those who survived or did not develop the outcome of interest) or "failure" (indicating those who died or developed the outcome of interest)" during the study period. The minimum information needed to calculate the sample size for a randomized controlled trial includes:

a) Desired level of significance;
b) Desired study power;
c) Proportion of outcome anticipated in the comparison (standard treatment or placebo) group; and
d) Desired treatment difference.

Given all the above information, one can calculate the sample size for a clinical trial by using the following formula (Formula 17.18) [8]:

$$n = \frac{P_1\left(100 - P_1\right) + P_2\left(100 - P_2\right)}{\left(P_2 - P_1\right)^2} \times \left(Z_{\alpha/2} + Z_\beta\right)^2 \qquad \left[\text{Formula } 17.18\right]$$

Where

- n is the required sample size in each group;
- P_1 is the percentage of success in the standard treatment group;
- P_2 is the percentage of success expected in the other (new) treatment group;
- α is the desired level of significance for the detection of the difference in treatment outcome;
- β is the Type II error, while $(1 - \beta)$ is the power of the study; and
- $Z_{\alpha/2}$ and Z_β are the values from the standard normal distribution (Z-distribution) corresponding to the specified values of α (two-sided) and β.

Example
A randomized double-blind study is designed to evaluate the effectiveness of aspirin in preventing mortality among patients with ischemic heart disease (IHD). It has been decided that the comparison group will receive a placebo. The outcome of interest is the death of IHD patients due to myocardial infarction (MI) within two years of treatment. Published data indicate that approximately 18% of IHD patients die within two years due to MI. It is hypothesized (anticipated) that aspirin will reduce the mortality rate by at least 20% (i.e., 20% of 18%) compared to placebo. If researchers want to detect this treatment difference at a 5% level of significance and 90% power, how many IHD patients need to be enrolled in the study?

From the example above, we have the following information:

- P_1 is 18.0%;
- P_2 is 14.4% (a 20% reduction from 18.0%);
- α is 5% or 0.05 [$Z_{\alpha/2}$ is 1.96; obtained from Table 17.2 (for a two-sided test)]; and
- Power $(1 - \beta)$ is 90% (Z_β is 1.28; obtained from Table 17.2)

The sample size needed for the study is 2,194 IHD patients in each group (i.e., 2,194 IHD patients in the aspirin group and 2,194 IHD patients in the placebo group).

17.5.2 Sample Size When the Outcome Measure Is a Mean (Quantitative Outcome)

In some clinical trials, the outcome measurement for patients is quantitative. The sample size for such outcome measures can be calculated using the following formula (Formula 17.19) [8]:

$$n = \frac{2\sigma^2}{\left(\mu_2 - \mu_1\right)^2} \times (Z_{\alpha/2} + Z_\beta)^2 \qquad \left[\text{Formula 17.19}\right]$$

Where

- n is the required sample size in each group;
- μ_1 is the mean response in the standard treatment group;
- μ_2 is the anticipated mean response in the other treatment group;
- α is the desired level of significance for the detection of the difference in treatment outcome;
- β is the Type II error, while $(1 - \beta)$ is the power of the study; and
- $Z_{\alpha/2}$ and Z_β are the values from the standard normal distribution (Z-distribution) corresponding to the specified values of α (two-sided) and β.

Example

An evaluation of iron supplementation during pregnancy for the prevention of low birthweight (LBW) is planned. Researchers will randomly assign pregnant women to either an iron or a placebo group. The birthweight of newborn infants will be the principal measure of treatment response. Published studies indicate that the mean birthweight of newborn infants of untreated pregnant women (i.e., pregnant women who did not take iron tablets) is 2,500 g, with a standard deviation of 700 g. It is anticipated that iron supplementation during pregnancy will increase the mean birthweight by at least 375 g (a 15% increase in birthweight). The independent samples t-test will be used to determine the significance of the difference at a 5% level of significance. If the power of the study is set at 80%, how many pregnant women will be required for the study?

From the example above, we have the following information for calculating the sample size:

- μ_1 is 2,500 g;
- μ_2 is 2,875 g (2,500 + 375);
- σ is 700 g;
- α is 5% or 0.05 [$Z_{\alpha/2}$ is 1.96; obtained from Table 17.2 (for a two-sided test)]; and
- Power $(1 - \beta)$ is 80% (Z_β is 0.84; obtained from Table 17.2).

Using Formula 17.19, one can easily calculate the sample size. The minimum sample size required for the study is 55 pregnant women in each group (i.e., 55 pregnant women in the iron supplementation group and 55 pregnant women in the placebo group).

17.5.3 Unequal Treatment Allocation in Clinical Trials

Unequal treatment allocation is sometimes planned due to ethical concerns. For example, for a clinical trial in severely ill patients, it may be ethically desirable to have more subjects in the new treatment group (assumed to be superior to the other treatment) than in the standard treatment or placebo group.

When an unequal treatment allocation is planned, with more subjects in one arm than in the other, the following formulas (Formulas 17.20 and 17.21) can be used to adjust the sample size. If n is the desired sample size calculated using Formula 17.18 or 17.19, then the sample sizes for each arm are given by [9]:

$$\text{Sample size, n1} = \frac{n}{2} \times (1+k) \qquad \left[\text{Formula 17.20}\right]$$

$$\text{Sample size, n2} = \frac{n}{2} \times \left(1+\frac{1}{k}\right) \qquad \left[\text{Formula 17.21}\right]$$

Where

- n1 is the sample size for the first arm;

- n2 is the sample size for second arm; and

- k is the allocation ratio (n1 ÷ n2).

For example, consider a trial with an unequal allocation ratio of 2:1 between Arm1 and Arm2. If the sample size (n) calculated using Formula 17.18 is 2,194, the trial needs 3,291 subjects in Arm1 and 1,646 in Arm2.

References

1.   Daniel WW. *Biostatistics: A Foundation for Analysis in the Health Sciences.* 7th ed. India: Wiley; 1999.

2.   Sullivan LM. *Essentials of Biostatistics in Public Health*. 3rd ed. Burlington: Jones & Bartlett Learning; 2018.

3.   Lwanga SK, Lemeshow S. *Sample Size Determination in Health Studies: A Practical Manual*. Geneva: World Health Organization; 1991.

4.   World Health Organization. *Calculation of sample size for a single cross-sectional cluster survey*; 2023. Available from: https://mnsurvey.nutritionintl.org/categories/13

5.   Naing L, Winn T, Rusli BN. Practical issues in calculating the sample size for prevalence studies. *Arch Orofac Sci*. 2006;1:9–14.

6.   Schlesselman JJ, Stolley PD. *Case-Control Studies: Design, Conduct, Analysis*. Oxford: Oxford University Press; 1982.

7.   Chandrasekaran S, Sreedharan J, Gopakumar A. Sample size estimation in cohort studies for testing of relative risk. *Int J Sci Technol Res*. 2020;9(2):5552–8.

8.   Pocock SJ. *Clinical Trials: A Practical Approach*. New York: Wiley; 1984.

9.   Sakpal TV. Sample size estimation in clinical trial. *Perspect Clin Res*. 2010;1(2):67–9. PubMed PMID: 21829786; PMCID: PMC3148614.

18

Sampling Methods

Mohammad Tajul Islam

The main purpose of data collection is to learn about a population. In research, drawing valid conclusions about a population relies heavily on the sampling method and sample size. Sampling is the process of selecting a subset of individuals, groups, or elements from a larger population to draw inferences about the whole.

The quality of research depends on the quality of sampling and data collection. Before deciding on the sampling method, one should define the study population. The type of sampling method to be employed for a study depends on the study objectives, available resources, logic, and judgment.

Usually, the population is too large for most studies. A small but carefully chosen sample is not only manageable in terms of cost and time but can effectively represent the population. The purpose of sampling is to provide a valid estimate of a population parameter and to test hypotheses in the study [1]. In this chapter, the fundamental principles and sampling techniques, which are integral to ensuring the validity and generalizability of research findings, have been discussed.

18.1 Why Is a Sample Preferred Over Studying the Whole Population?

A sample is a subset (a part) of a population, and it may or may not be representative. A representative sample is a sample where individuals in the sample reflect the characteristics of the entire population from which it is drawn. In research, a representative sample is preferred because it reflects the important characteristics (such as age, gender, socioeconomic status, or other relevant factors) of the entire population, making the results generalizable. The representativeness of a sample primarily depends on how the sample

DOI: 10.1201/9781003654803-18

is drawn and its size. A representative sample should be selected randomly, and its size should be determined using standard statistical methods.

Sampling is a practical, cost-effective, and efficient method that allows researchers to collect detailed and accurate data to draw valid conclusions about a population without the need to study every individual within it. Studying a sample over the entire population is preferred for several reasons [4]:

> *Cost and time efficiency:* Collecting data from an entire population can be prohibitively expensive and time-consuming. Sampling allows researchers to gather the necessary information at a minimum cost and time. A well-selected sample can provide valid estimates without requiring data collection from the entire population over an extended period. Additionally, collecting data from an entire population requires significant resources, such as personnel, equipment, and logistical support. Sampling optimizes the use of available resources.

> *Practicality:* In many situations, it is impractical or even impossible to reach every individual in a population for data collection. Sampling offers a feasible alternative that can still provide valid and reliable information.

> *Manageability:* Data collection from a sample requires fewer human resources and allows researchers greater control over fieldwork. In contrast, managing the large volume of data collected from an entire population can be cumbersome and challenging. A small sample size makes data collection, processing, and analysis more manageable and reduces the likelihood of errors.

> *Accuracy:* Detailed and accurate information can be collected from a sample, which is difficult to achieve when studying the entire population.

> *Ethical considerations:* In certain studies, particularly those addressing sensitive topics or involving vulnerable populations, it is often considered more ethical to restrict data collection to a sample to minimize potential harm.

18.2 Sampling Frame and Sampling Unit

A sampling frame is a complete list of all members (study subjects, elements, or units) of the population from which the sample is to be drawn. The sampling frame is the basis for drawing a sample [7]. It serves as a tool to ensure that every member of the population has a chance to be included in the sample. The sampling frame should be up-to-date and free from omissions and duplications. Any omissions or duplications in the sampling frame can introduce bias and affect the validity of the research findings.

A distinct and identifiable unit (such as an individual or a group of individuals) of a population for drawing a sample is called the sampling unit. It is the smallest entity from which data are collected. Sometimes, a sampling unit is also called an element. The nature of the sampling unit can vary depending on the study design and objectives. For instance, a sampling unit can be an individual person, a household, an organization, or any other entity relevant to the research objective.

18.3 Sampling and Non-Sampling Errors

Data from sample surveys are subject to both sampling and non-sampling errors. Sampling error (or random error) is the difference between the sample value or statistic (such as the sample mean or proportion) and the corresponding population parameter, such as the true mean or proportion of the entire population [1]. Sampling error is linked to the sample size and the method used to draw the sample. Although it cannot be completely eliminated, even with proper sampling techniques, it can be minimized by using a sufficiently large sample, specifically calculated for the study, and employing an appropriate sampling design.

The other term "sampling variation" refers to the variability in sample statistics (such as sample means or proportions) that arises from drawing multiple samples of the same size from the same population.

On the contrary, non-sampling error refers to all sources of error that can occur in a study, apart from those related to the sampling design. These errors can arise from various sources. The common sources of non-sampling errors are: a) improper specification of the study population; b) inaccurate or incomplete sampling frame; c) faulty method of sample selection; d) faulty method of data collection; e) biased survey questionnaire; f) measurement errors; g) nonresponse; and h) lack of supervision of fieldwork and data processing.

When designing and conducting a study, it is important to minimize both sampling and non-sampling errors to ensure accurate results as much as possible.

18.4 Sampling with and Without Replacement

Sampling can be done with or without replacement [1]. In sampling with replacement, a sampling unit or individual is drawn from the population, observed, and then returned to the population before another unit or individual is selected. This means that a unit or individual has a chance to be selected more than once in the sample. This sampling technique is often used in theoretical studies, bootstrapping, and simulations.

On the other hand, in sampling without replacement, once a unit or individual is selected from the population and observed, it is not returned to the population for subsequent selection of units or individuals. This approach ensures that each unit or individual can be selected only once in the sample. Sampling without replacement is more efficient and is primarily used for practical applications, such as surveys and other studies.

18.5 Sampling Methods

Sampling is a scientific method used in research to select study subjects or units from a target population. Sampling techniques commonly used in research can be classified as: a) probability sampling methods and b) nonprobability sampling methods [2–7].

Each method has its own strengths and limitations. The choice of an appropriate sampling technique depends on the research objectives, the nature of the population, and the available resources. For instance, probability sampling methods are valued for their ability to support statistical inference, while non-probability sampling methods are often utilized for their practicality and capacity to provide deeper insights in exploratory research.

18.5.1 Probability Sampling Methods

Probability sampling is based on the principle of random selection of study subjects. In probability sampling, each unit in the population has a known (non-zero) probability of being selected. One key advantage of probability sampling is that sampling errors can be calculated. In nonprobability sampling, the degree to which the sample differs from the population remains unknown. The following are the approaches to probability sampling methods:

1) Simple random sampling;
2) Systematic random sampling;
3) Stratified random sampling; and
4) Cluster sampling.

18.5.1.1 *Simple Random Sampling*

Simple random sampling is the purest form of probability sampling, where each member of the population has an equal and known chance of being selected. A sampling frame is required before drawing a simple random sample. When the population size is very large, it is often difficult or impossible to identify every member of the population to create the sampling frame. In such situations, this type of sampling may not be feasible.

A simple random sample can be drawn from a population using random numbers. These random numbers can be generated using a random number table, calculator, or computer. To draw a simple random sample, each member or unit of the population is first assigned a unique number (identification number). Then, using the random number table or computer-generated random numbers, members are selected for the sample.

A simple random sample is easy to draw and is the basis for all other sampling techniques. It is particularly suitable when the population is homogeneous about the characteristic of interest. However, the disadvantages of the simple random sampling method are:

- A sampling frame is required, making it time-consuming and costly, especially if the population is large;

- The sample may include very high or very low values if the population is not homogeneous; and

- If the population is large, selected units may be spread out across the population, making data collection difficult, time-consuming, and costly.

18.5.1.2 *Systematic Random Sampling*

Systematic random sampling is often used as an alternative to simple random sampling. It is a modified form of the simple random sampling method. A sampling frame is usually needed to draw this type of sample. In this method, the first unit (or subject) of the population is selected using the simple random sampling method, and subsequent units are then selected at fixed intervals. The steps for selecting a systematic random sample include:

- Develop a sampling frame with unique identification (ID) numbers for each unit (or subject) in the population;

- Calculate the sampling interval by dividing the total population size by the sample size calculated for the study;

- Select the first unit from the population using the simple random sampling method from the first sampling interval; and

- Finally, select subsequent units at fixed intervals based on the calculated sampling interval.

For example, if you want to select 20 patients out of 100 in a hospital, first make a sampling frame by assigning unique identification (ID) numbers to all 100 patients. The sampling interval, in this case, is 5 (100 ÷ 20). Next, select the first patient using the simple random sampling method from the ID numbers between one and five. Suppose the first patient selected has the ID number two. The subsequent patients to be selected will have ID numbers 7 (2 + 5), 12 (7 + 5), 17 (12 + 5), and so on (i.e., every fifth patient after selecting the first one).

The advantages of systematic random sampling over the simple random sampling technique are its simplicity (easy to select), selected units are evenly distributed across the entire population, and sampling is possible even when a sampling frame cannot be prepared.

18.5.1.3 Stratified Random Sampling

Stratified random sampling is a widely used probability sampling technique that is considered superior to simple random sampling, as it reduces sampling error. In this method, the study population is divided into two or more homogeneous subgroups (or strata) based on one or more characteristics of the study subjects. A stratum is a subset (subgroup) of a population that shares at least one common characteristic. For example, based on the area of residence, a study population can be divided into urban and rural populations. In this case, urban and rural areas serve as strata, with each stratum being homogeneous in terms of its area of residence. Other examples of strata include males and females or slum and non-slum areas.

Once the study population is stratified, a desired number of study subjects (elements) are randomly selected from each stratum using techniques such as simple random sampling or systematic random sampling. This method is particularly suitable when the study population is heterogeneous with respect to a characteristic of interest, such as contraceptive prevalence rates in urban and rural areas. Stratified random sampling ensures representation of all groups within the population. Other advantages of this method are that it is easy to apply and produces more accurate statistical results.

The number of elements (subjects) selected from the strata can be either *proportionate or disproportionate*. Therefore, researchers need to determine the actual representation (percentage) of each stratum within the target population before taking a sample. In proportionate sampling (the ideal approach), the sample size allocated to each stratum corresponds to the size of the stratum relative to the entire population. For instance, in Bangladesh, the urban and rural populations constitute 40% and 60%, respectively. If researchers plan to conduct a study involving rural and urban populations with a proportionate sample size of 500 women of reproductive age, they should select 40% (200) of the women from urban areas and 60% (300) of the women from rural areas. In contrast, disproportionate sampling does not maintain this ratio.

Stratified random sampling is often used when one or more strata in the population exhibit a low (or high) prevalence of a condition (such as a disease or other health problems) compared to other strata. The main features of the stratified random sampling method are:

- The population is divided into a number of sub-groups, known as strata;
- All individuals within a strata are homogeneous with respect to at least one characteristic;
- A sample is drawn independently from each stratum;
- This method provides better estimation of population parameters; and
- Estimates can be obtained for various subgroups within the population.

18.5.1.4 Cluster Sampling

A cluster is a group or collection of similar elements within a larger population. Cluster sampling is a probability sampling technique in which researchers divide the study population into several groups or clusters. Researchers then randomly select one or more clusters to include in the sample, using methods such as simple random sampling or systematic random sampling. In cluster sampling, clusters are selected in such a way that each cluster looks like a mini population. This method is commonly used when it is impractical or too costly to sample individuals directly from the entire population.

Each cluster should ideally be heterogeneous internally but homogeneous externally, meaning that the elements within each cluster should be diverse, while the clusters themselves should be similar to one another. Cluster sampling helps data collection by reducing costs and logistical challenges, while still providing a representative sample of the population. However, an important disadvantage of this method is that the sampling error tends to be higher in cluster sampling compared to simple random sampling.

The main difference between stratified random sampling and cluster sampling is that in stratified random sampling, elements are selected from all strata, whereas in cluster sampling, elements are only selected from some of the clusters.

For example, if a researcher wants to estimate the prevalence of asthma in a district but cannot use simple or systematic random sampling due to the unavailability or high cost of constructing a sampling frame, cluster sampling becomes a suitable alternative. This method allows for sampling with minimal cost and time.

To take a cluster sample, first, group the study population in the district into clusters, such as unions, wards, or villages. Then, use either simple random sampling or systematic random sampling to select a number of clusters for the study. Afterward, select all or a portion (sample) of the study subjects (elements) from each selected cluster for data collection. The main features of cluster sampling are:

- The population is divided into clusters of homogeneous units, usually based on geographic proximity;
- A sample of clusters is then selected; and
- All units (or elements) or a sample of units from the chosen clusters are selected for data collection.

Cluster sampling can be classified into single-stage (or one-stage), two-stage, and multistage cluster sampling, depending on the number of stages involved in obtaining the sample. In most cases, cluster sampling follows multiple stages, where each stage represents a step taken to obtain the desired sample.

Single-stage cluster sampling
In single-stage cluster sampling, as the name suggests, sampling is done in a single step. For example, if you want to determine the proportion of women delivered by skilled providers in a district and consider villages as your clusters, you should first select the desired number of villages (clusters) from all the villages in the district. Then, collect data from all elements (eligible women) within each selected cluster (village) for your study.

Two-stage Cluster Sampling
In single-stage cluster sampling, all elements (study subjects) from the selected clusters are included in the study. In two-stage cluster sampling, instead of selecting all elements from the chosen clusters, a subset (sample) of elements is selected from each cluster using either simple random sampling or systematic random sampling techniques. In this approach, the first stage is the selection of clusters, and the second stage is the selection of elements from the selected clusters using the simple or systematic random sampling method.

Multistage cluster sampling
Multistage, or multiple-stage, cluster sampling extends beyond two-stage cluster sampling by adding one or more additional steps to select study subjects. In multistage cluster sampling, clusters are selected randomly (either by simple random sampling or systematic random sampling) in different stages until the final sampling cluster is reached. In this method, larger clusters of the population are divided into smaller clusters through several stages, and clusters are selected progressively from larger to smaller at each stage.

For example, to determine the prevalence of diabetes among adults in a division (province), a researcher may first select one or more districts from the division (first stage). Next, one or more upazilas (sub-districts) are selected from each selected district (second stage), followed by the selection of one or more villages from each upazila (third stage). Finally, all eligible individuals from the selected villages are included in the study.

18.5.2 Nonprobability Sampling Methods

Nonprobability sampling is a sampling technique in which the sample is drawn from the target population based on specific criteria rather than using a random selection method. In this approach, the sample is selected according to the researcher's convenience, expertise, or judgment. The probability of each unit in the population being selected for the sample is unknown. Nonprobability sampling often results in biased sample selection, which is a significant limitation, particularly in quantitative studies. Nonprobability sampling methods include:

1) Convenience sampling;
2) Purposive or judgmental sampling;
3) Quota sampling; and
4) Snowball sampling.

18.5.2.1 Convenience Sampling

Convenience sampling is a nonprobability sampling method commonly used in clinical, exploratory, or pilot studies. As the name suggests, the sample is selected based on the researchers' convenience, such as ease of accessibility. This method is particularly useful in preliminary research efforts to obtain rough estimates of results without incurring the cost or time required for taking a random sample. For instance, it may be employed in pilot studies or for pre-testing a questionnaire. In clinical trials, convenience sampling is often used to select study subjects based on their availability and accessibility.

18.5.2.2 Purposive or Judgmental Sampling

Purposive or judgmental sampling is a widely used nonprobability sampling method. In this approach, the researchers select the sample based on their judgment. It is an extension of the convenience sampling technique. For example, a researcher may, based on experience, decide to study one brothel (out of many) to assess socio-demographic characteristics, condom use, STI prevalence, and other factors influencing transmission of HIV infection. However, when employing this method, the researcher must be confident that the selected site is reasonably representative of other brothels. Other examples of purposive sampling include selecting participants for key informant interviews (KII) and in-depth interviews (IDIs) in qualitative studies.

18.5.2.3 Quota Sampling

Quota sampling is a nonprobability sampling method that resembles stratified random sampling. In this approach, the researcher first identifies the strata and their proportions, as represented in the population, similar to stratified random sampling. However, instead of selecting study subjects randomly from each stratum, as in stratified sampling, convenience or judgmental sampling is used to select the required number of study subjects from each stratum.

The basic difference between quota sampling and stratified sampling lies in the selection process. In stratified sampling, subjects are selected randomly from each stratum, whereas in quota sampling, subjects are selected purposively or based on convenience from each stratum.

18.5.2.4 Snowball Sampling

Snowball sampling, also known as chain sampling or sequential sampling, is a nonprobability sampling technique. This approach of sampling is used when the target population is rare or difficult to reach through traditional sampling methods, such as street-based sex workers, drug users, or undocumented immigrants. This method relies on referrals from initial subjects to identify and recruit additional participants, creating a "snowball" effect as the sample grows.

In snowball sampling, the researcher first identifies and selects a few initial participants (study subjects) who possess the desired characteristics (e.g., injecting drug users). These initial participants are interviewed, and at the end of each interview, they are asked to refer other individuals they know who meet the study criteria. These referrals form the basis for subsequent rounds of sampling. The process continues iteratively until the desired sample size is achieved.

References

1.   Daniel WW. *Biostatistics: A Foundation for Analysis in the Health Sciences.* 7th ed. India: Wiley; 1999.
2.   Bhardwaj P. Types of sampling in research. *J Pract Cardiovasc Sci.* 2019;5:157–63.

3. Taherdoost H. Sampling methods in research methodology; how to choose a sampling technique for research. *Int J Acad Res Manag*. 2016;5(2):18–27.

4. Makwana D, Engineer P, Dabhi A, Chudasama H. Sampling methods in research: A review. *Int J Trend Sci Res Dev*. 2023;7(3):762–68. Available from: www.ijtsrd.com/papers/ijtsrd57470.pdf

5. Mulisa F. Sampling techniques involving human subjects: Applications, pitfalls, and suggestions for further studies. *Int J Acad Res Educ*. 2022;8(1):75–84.

6. Elfil M, Negida A. Sampling methods in clinical research; an educational review. *Emerg (Tehran)*. 2017;5(1):e52.

7. Obilor EI. Convenience and purposive sampling techniques: Are they the same? *Int J Innov Soc Sci Educ Res*. 2023;11(1):1–7.

19

Application of Artificial Intelligence in Public Health

Russell Kabir

Epidemiological research is crucial for understanding disease dynamics, identifying risk factors, and informing public health interventions. Traditional epidemiological approaches often face challenges when dealing with large and complex datasets and slow decision-making processes. Artificial intelligence (AI) offers the potential to enhance epidemiological research by improving data processing, analytical capabilities, and evidence-based decision-making [1]. This chapter presents an overview of the application of AI in public health, focusing on digital surveillance methods, real-world data applications, and the emerging field of climate change epidemiology.

19.1 AI in Public Health: Applications and Methods

AI is being applied to various aspects of public health, including disease surveillance, outbreak prediction, risk assessment, and intervention strategies [1–3]. Machine learning (ML), a subtype of AI, enables computers to learn from data without explicit programming, draw conclusions, and improve disease prediction and patient care [4, 5]. Below, some evidence-based uses of AI in the field of epidemiology and public health are provided.

19.1.1 Disease Surveillance

Digital epidemiology, which uses data generated outside traditional public health systems, has been employed for disease surveillance for over two decades [6, 7]. The increasing volume of potentially useful data from social media and other big data streams has further enhanced digital surveillance efforts. AI-driven systems can analyze this data to provide early warnings and rapid responses to outbreaks [7].

DOI: 10.1201/9781003654803-19

19.1.2 Early Detection and Monitoring

AI systems like EPIWATCH can provide early signals of outbreaks before official authorities are aware [3]. These systems are crucial because infectious diseases often exhibit exponential growth, causing rapid surges in cases that can overwhelm healthcare infrastructure. Traditional surveillance methods, which rely on laboratory reporting and validation, can be substantially delayed compared to AI-driven approaches [3]. For example, HealthMap is responsive to specific emergencies, such as providing a monkeypox (Mpox) dashboard in 2022 [3].

19.1.3 Open-Source Data

The use of open-source data is essential for timely epidemic intelligence [3]. Several quantitative and automated internet-based systems have been developed, but many remain niche tools due to paywalls or restricted access. To effectively prevent future pandemics, AI-based technologies need to be widely and easily accessible, embedded within public health departments, and supported by adequate training [3]. For example, one of the earliest systems, ProMED-Mail, relies on doctors and professionals to report outbreaks and remains an important qualitative system [3]. Another example is EPIWATCH, which offers open access to its data and provides a global map and table with visualization options. It also includes tools for seasonal forecasting and determining the origins of epidemics [3].

19.1.4 Predictive Modelling

AI algorithms can be used for predictive modelling, which is crucial for forecasting disease trends and informing public health interventions [2]. These models can identify high-risk populations, predict disease spread, and evaluate the effectiveness of interventions [5]. Machine learning (ML) and deep learning (DL) have been employed in early detection, monitoring, and prediction of future outbreaks. These techniques can also aid in the development of drugs and vaccines [8]. AI has been used to monitor and detect potential outbreaks and assess associated risks, offering new hope for transforming public health practices [9].

19.1.5 COVID-19 Surveillance

During the COVID-19 pandemic, AI played a significant role in surveillance, case reporting, contact tracing, and public health monitoring. Traditional tracking methods were replaced by intelligent solutions using smartphones, portable devices, and drones, which produce large amounts of data that need to be processed instantly [10].

19.1.6 Data Analytics and Visualization

AI enhances data analytics and visualization, enabling public health officials to gain insights from complex datasets and communicate findings effectively [2].

19.1.7 Geographic Information Systems

AI, combined with a geographical information system (GIS), can be used for geo-location and visualization of epidemic data. This allows for the identification of spatial patterns and the monitoring of disease spread in specific geographic areas [9].

19.1.8 Digital Media and Data Collection

Digital media, the Internet of Things (IoT), blockchain, and wearable devices play a role in collecting surveillance data. Predictive modelling, image recognition, and GIS revolutionize disease detection, outbreak prediction, and resource allocation [2].

19.2 AI in Climate Change Epidemiology

Climate change significantly impacts human health by altering patterns of ambient exposures and disasters, including extreme temperatures, heat waves, wildfires, droughts, and floods [11, 12]. Climate epidemiology plays a vital role in informing policy related to these threats [11]. Climate change affects health through direct pathways, such as heat and cold effects on mortality, and indirect pathways, such as changes in vector-borne disease transmission and food security [12]. Populations in low and middle-income countries are particularly vulnerable to the health impacts of climate change due to higher exposures and lower adaptive capacities [13]. Climate change is leading to the geographical expansion of mosquitoes and other vectors, increasing the risk of diseases like dengue, malaria, and chikungunya [14]. AI can be used to model and predict the health impacts of climate change, identify vulnerable populations, and inform adaptation and mitigation strategies [15].

19.3 Real-World Data Applications and Examples

Mortality risk assessment
A machine-learning study using data from 83,227 hospital admissions to identify causes of influenza-like illnesses and assess risk factors for severe disease

and mortality. The study demonstrated that decision-tree analysis models were comparable to deep neural networks in predicting disease severity [16].

COVID-19 pandemic
AI-based surveillance and contact tracing were used in countries like Saudi Arabia to monitor and control the spread of COVID-19. These applications included smartphones, portable devices, and drones to collect and process data [10].

Vaccine distribution and access
During the COVID-19 pandemic, AI systems helped streamline vaccine production, supply chain management, distribution channels, and data collection based on geographical and demographic characteristics, addressing vaccine access inequality issues observed by WHO and IMF [17].

Diagnosis and treatment
AI has been used to analyze medical images (CT scans, X-rays) to diagnose COVID-19 and predict disease progression [18].

Disease transmission analysis
An AI-based random forest model was used for threshold-classification tasks to identify upward trend signals for extreme events in disease spread, achieving an average performance score of 0.880 in identifying emerging outbreaks [19].

Wastewater-based epidemiology
Wastewater-based epidemiology (WBE) is a tool that monitors the spread of infectious diseases and antimicrobial resistance at the community level by analyzing pooled wastewater [20].

Vector-borne diseases
AI can be used to model and predict the spread of vector-borne diseases like West Nile virus, considering climate and environmental factors [21].

Lung cancer
AI applications in lung cancer include epidemiology (prevention and screening), diagnosis by X-rays, computed tomography (CT), positron emission tomography (PET), and biomarker detection; and treatment planning [22].

Colorectal cancer
AI can aid in the epidemiology of colorectal cancer through methods like GeoAI and digital epidemiology. It can also improve diagnostic tools and treatment approaches [23].

Data integration
Combining multiple data types (e.g., clinical, environmental, and social) can enhance the accuracy and comprehensiveness of AI models [24].

Life-course epidemiology
Integrating AI in life-course epidemiology can help understand the complex interplay between biological, social, and environmental factors that shape health trajectories across the lifespan [24].

Real-world evidence analytics
Saama's real-world analytics is a cloud-based application that helps life sciences companies monitor large populations during clinical trials and forecast disease incidence or prevalence using machine learning. The system was trained on billions of patients' electronic medical records to predict treatment patterns and disease prevalence [25].

References

1. Li Y, Zou Y, Xu H. From data to decisions: The integration of AI in epidemiological research. *Front Comput Intell Syst.* 2024;9:23–9. https://doi.org/10.54097/7jktck77

2. Reinoso GPG, Haro HDP, Madero JLA, Escaleras LGO, Quinquiguano MIA, Pilatasig WJM, et al. Epidemiological surveillance innovative applications for community and public health: A systematic review. *Int J Med Sci Clin Res Stud.* 2024;4(3).

3. MacIntyre CR, Lim S, Quigley A. Preventing the next pandemic: Use of artificial intelligence for epidemic monitoring and alerts. *Cell Rep Med.* 2022;3:100867. https://doi.org/10.1016/j.xcrm.2022.100867

4. Bini SA. Artificial intelligence, machine learning, deep learning, and cognitive computing: What do these terms mean and how will they impact health care? *J Arthroplasty.* 2018;33:2358–61. https://doi.org/10.1016/j.arth.2018.02.067

5. Habehh H, Gohel S. Machine learning in healthcare. *Curr Genomics.* 2021;22:291–300. https://doi.org/10.2174/1389202922666210705124359

6. Mello MM, Wang CJ. Ethics and governance for digital disease surveillance. *Science.* 2020;368:951–4. https://doi.org/10.1126/science.abb9045

7. Kostkova P. Disease surveillance data sharing for public health: The next ethical frontiers. *Life Sci Soc Policy.* 2018;14:16. https://doi.org/10.1186/s40504-018-0078-x

8. Addaali B, Latif R, Saddik A. Addressing the spread of infectious diseases in the era of explainable AI. *2024 World Conference on Complex Systems (WCCS),* IEEE; 2024:1–6. https://doi.org/10.1109/WCCS62745.2024.10765539

9. Jia JS, Lu X, Yuan Y, Xu G, Jia J, Christakis NA. Population flow drives spatio-temporal distribution of COVID-19 in China. *Nature.* 2020;582:389–94. https://doi.org/10.1038/s41586-020-2284-y

10. Dawood AS, Dawood A, Dawood S. Catatonia after COVID-19 infection: Scoping review. *BJPsych Bull.* 2023;47:208–19. https://doi.org/10.1192/bjb.2022.30

11. Anderson GB, Barnes EA, Bell ML, Dominici F. The future of climate epidemiology: Opportunities for advancing health research in the context of

climate change. *Am J Epidemiol.* 2019;188:866–72. https://doi.org/10.1093/aje/kwz034

12. Kabir R, Khan HTA, Ball E, Caldwell K. Climate change and public health situations in the Coastal Areas of Bangladesh. *Int J Soc Sci Stud.* 2014;2. https://doi.org/10.11114/ijsss.v2i3.426

13. Sauerborn R. A gaping research gap regarding the climate change impact on health in poor countries. *Eur J Epidemiol.* 2017;32:855–6. https://doi.org/10.1007/s10654-017-0258-7

14. George AM, Ansumana R, de Souza DK, Niyas VKM, Zumla A, Bockarie MJ. Climate change and the rising incidence of vector-borne diseases globally. *Int J Infect Dis.* 2024;139:143–5. https://doi.org/10.1016/j.ijid.2023.12.004

15. YesuJyothi Y, Shaik S, Venkateswarlu Y. Enhancing climate analysis with integrated data and transparent AI methods via Stochastic processes. *2024 8th International Conference on I-SMAC (IoT in Social, Mobile, Analytics and Cloud) (I-SMAC)*, IEEE; 2024:1570–6. https://doi.org/10.1109/I-SMAC61858.2024.10714600

16. Parums DV. Editorial: Infectious disease surveillance using artificial intelligence (AI) and its role in epidemic and pandemic preparedness. *Med Sci Moni.* 2023;29. https://doi.org/10.12659/MSM.941209

17. Anjaria P, Asediya V, Bhavsar P, Pathak A, Desai D, Patil V. Artificial intelligence in public health: Revolutionizing epidemiological surveillance for pandemic preparedness and equitable vaccine access. *Vaccines (Basel).* 2023;11:1154. https://doi.org/10.3390/vaccines11071154

18. Syeda HB, Syed M, Sexton KW, Syed S, Begum S, Syed F, et al. Role of machine learning techniques to Tackle the COVID-19 crisis: Systematic review. *JMIR Med Inform.* 2021;9:e23811. https://doi.org/10.2196/23811

19. Melchane S, Elmir Y, Kacimi F, Boubchir L. Artificial intelligence for infectious disease prediction and prevention: A comprehensive review. *Acta U Sapien Inform.* 2025;16:160–97. https://doi.org/10.47745/ausi-2024-0010

20. Sim MR. The COVID-19 pandemic: Major risks to healthcare and other workers on the front line. *Occup Environ Med.* 2020;77:281. https://doi.org/10.1136/oemed-2020-106567

21. Heidecke J, Lavarello Schettini A, Rocklöv J. West Nile virus eco-epidemiology and climate change. *PLOS Clim.* 2023;2:e0000129. https://doi.org/10.1371/journal.pclm.0000129

22. Kotoulas S-C, Spyratos D, Porpodis K, Domvri K, Boutou A, Kaimakamis E, et al. A thorough review of the clinical applications of artificial intelligence in lung cancer. *Cancers (Basel).* 2025;17:882. https://doi.org/10.1038/s41467-021-26643-8

23. Yu G, Sun K, Xu C, Shi X-H, Wu C, Xie T, et al. Accurate recognition of colorectal cancer with semi-supervised deep learning on pathological images. *Nat Commun.* 2021;12:6311. https://doi.org/10.1038/s41467-021-26643-8

24. Chen F, Wang L , Hong J, Jiang J, Zhou L. Unmasking bias in artificial intelligence: A systematic review of bias detection and mitigation strategies in electronic health record-based models. *J Am Med Inform Assoc.* 2024;31:1172–83. https://doi.org/10.1093/jamia/ocae060

25. Jesus AN. Artificial intelligence in epidemiology – current use-cases. *EMERJ* 2019. https://emerj.com/artificial-intelligence-epidemiology/

20

Ethical Considerations in Epidemiological Research with Human Subjects

Mohammad Delwer Hossain Hawlader

I'm a good person. Why do I need to worry about ethics?

Research is an integral part of development. Epidemiological studies are conducted to generate evidence to improve human health. Due to technological advances, it is possible to quickly integrate and link various sources of data and analyze them. Given that epidemiological studies are carried out on human populations, safety, consent, privacy, confidentiality, and other issues are concerns. This chapter briefly describes the ethical and professional issues in relation to epidemiologic studies.

20.1 Ethical Considerations in Epidemiological Studies

"Ethical conduct" literally means simply doing the right thing, but in reality, it is more complex. It involves acting in the right spirit, out of an abiding respect and concern for one's fellow creatures. Epidemiological studies conducted with or about people, or their personal or physical data, should be conducted with the sole intention of doing good.

Epidemiological studies involve significant risks, and it is possible for things to go wrong. Despite the best of intentions and care in planning and practice, sometimes matters go awry; mishaps may arise because of technical errors or an ethical insensitivity, neglect, or disregard [1].

On rare occasions, the practice of research has even involved deliberate and appalling violations of human subjects. Earlier, in the 1900s, no regulations existed regarding the ethical use of human subjects in research. There were no guidelines or any code drawn out for conduct, and no Institutional Review Board (IRB).

DOI: 10.1201/9781003654803-20

20.2 Ethics and Law

Ethics is the science of morals. Ethics comprises guidelines and principles that inform people about how to live or how to behave in a particular situation. Research ethics are the set of ethical guidelines on how scientific research should be conducted and disseminated. Research ethics are the ethical principles that researchers must follow to protect the rights, dignity, and welfare of research participants. Ethics has no legal binding on the people. On the other hand, the law consists of a set of rules and regulations by the authority or government. Law creates a legally binding.

20.3 Historical Background of Human-Subject-Research

The current system of oversight and protection in human-subject-research has developed over the last five decades. The principles of conducting human research were first developed as the Nuremberg code following unethical Nazi research. The Nuremberg Code has three basic elements: a) voluntary informed consent, b) favourable risk/benefit analysis, and c) right to withdraw without repercussions, which became the foundation for subsequent ethical codes and research regulations.

In 1964, the World Medical Association released the Declaration of Helsinki, built on the principles of the Nuremberg Code. Numerous research improprieties between 1950 and 1974 in the US prompted Congressional deliberations about human-subject-research oversight. Congress's first legislation to protect the rights and welfare of human subjects was the National Research Act of 1974, which created the National Commission for Protection of Human Subjects of Biomedical and Behavioral Research and issued the Belmont Report. The Belmont Report stated the fundamental principles for conducting human-subjects research: a) respect for persons, b) beneficence, and c) justice. The Office of Human Research Protections oversees Title 45, Part 46 of the Code of Federal Regulations, which pertains to human-subjects research. That office indirectly oversees human-subjects research through local institutional review boards (IRB). Since their inception, the principles of conducting human research, IRBs, and the Code for Federal Regulations have all advanced substantially [2].

20.3.1 Nazi Research

In its concentration camps in the early to mid-1940s, during World War II, a series of Nazi human medical experiments were carried out on large numbers of prisoners, including children. Chief target populations were Romani, Sinti, ethnic Poles, Soviet, disabled Germans, and Jews from across Europe. Nazi physicians and their assistants forced prisoners to participate in the research. The participants did not willingly volunteer or give consent for the procedures. The experiments were conducted without anesthesia and resulted in deaths, trauma, disfigurement, or permanent disability. The Nuremberg Code was created in the aftermath of these discoveries of the camp experiments and the trials that followed, to address abuses committed by medical professionals during the Holocaust. The Nuremberg Code of 1947 included the principle of informed consent and required standards for research. Twenty-three researchers involved in inhuman trials were taken to court, of which seven were given death sentences, nine were imprisoned, and seven were acquitted.

20.3.2 The Tuskegee Syphilis Study (1932–1972)

One of the key turning points in the development of guidelines for ethical conduct in research was a project conducted by the US Public Health Service. Six hundred low-income, African American males, 400 of whom were infected with syphilis, were monitored for 40 years. Although free medical examinations were conducted, the subjects were not told about their disease. Even though a proven cure (penicillin) became available in the 1950s, the study continued until 1972, with participants being denied treatment. In some cases, when the subjects were diagnosed as having syphilis by other physicians, researchers intervened to prevent treatment. The study sparked off a wide-scale public outrage when it became publicly known, and the US government was forced to close it in 1973.

Due to the publicity from the Tuskegee Syphilis Study, a National Commission for the Protection of Human Subjects of Biomedical and Behavioral Research was formed in the US. The committee was in charge of identifying the basic ethical principles that should underlie the conduct of biomedical and behavioural research involving human subjects, and developing mandatory guidelines that should be followed. The Commission drafted the Belmont report, a foundational document for the ethics of human-subject research in the United States [3].

20.4 Rules and Regulations of Human Subject Research

20.4.1 The Nuremberg Code

A well-known chapter in the history of research with human subjects opened on 9 December 1946, with a US military tribunal's criminal proceedings against the aforementioned 23 leading German physicians and administrators for their willing participation in war crimes and crimes against humanity. Among the charges were that German physicians conducted medical experiments on thousands of concentration camp prisoners without their consent. Most of the subjects of these experiments died or were permanently crippled as a result.

As a direct result of the trial, the Nuremberg Code was established in 1948, stating that "The voluntary consent of the human subject is absolutely essential", making it clear that subjects should give consent and that the benefits of the research must outweigh the risks [4].

Although it did not carry the force of law, the Nuremberg Code was the first international document, which advocated voluntary participation and informed consent.

20.4.2 The Declaration of Helsinki

In 1964, the World Medical Association established recommendations guiding medical doctors in biomedical research involving human subjects. The declaration governs international research ethics and defines rules for "research combined with clinical care" and "non-therapeutic research". This Declaration of Helsinki was revised in 1975, 1983, 1989, 1996, and 2013, and is the basis for good clinical practices used today. The issues addressed in the declaration of Helsinki include:

- Research with humans should be based on the results from laboratory and animal experimentation;
- Research protocols should be reviewed by an independent committee prior to initiation;
- Informed consent from research participants is necessary;
- Research should be conducted by medically/scientifically qualified individuals; and
- Risks should not exceed benefits.

20.4.3 Belmont Report

The Belmont report was written by the National Commission for the Protection of Human Subjects of Biomedical and Behavioral Research. The Commission, created because of the National Research Act of 1974, was charged with identifying the basic ethical principles that should underlie the conduct of biomedical and behavioral research involving human subjects and developing guidelines to ensure that such research is conducted in accordance with those principles. Informed by monthly discussions that spanned nearly four years and an intensive four days of deliberation in 1976, the Commission published the Belmont report in 1979, which identifies basic ethical principles and guidelines that address ethical issues arising from the conduct of research with human subjects [5]. According to the report, the three basic ethical principles and their corresponding applications are: a) respect for person (treating participants with respect and dignity, such as protection from abuse, privacy, and non-discrimination), b) beneficence (maximizing possible benefits and minimizing possible harms to participants), and c) justice (treating participants equally, ensuring equitable recruitment and selection of participants, and distributing benefits and burdens fairly).

20.5 Research on Human Subjects

Data regarding the living individual(s) the investigator (whether professional or student) is researching is obtained through intervention or interaction with the individual or with identifiable private information. Examples of research without living human subjects include programme evaluation or the analysis of data (or specimens) from the deceased. The associated principals and some areas of research ethics with human subjects are summarized in Box 20.1.

20.5.1 Integrity

The ultimate objective of epidemiology is to improve human health through disease prevention and improvement of disease outcome. Epidemiological studies involve human subjects, and commonly, the subjects who participate in research studies do not receive any personal benefits. Epidemiological

---

BOX 20.1   PRINCIPLES AND AREAS OF RESEARCH ETHICS

Principles:

- Integrity
- Voluntary participation
- No harm to the subjects
- Informed consent
- Anonymity

- Privacy
- Confidentiality
- Beneficence
- Dignity

Some research ethics:

- Research misconduct (falsification, fabrication and plagiarism)
- Collaboration issues (authorship, data ownership and management)
- Peer review

- Conflicts of interest or obligation
- Complicity and funding sources
- Animal subject research
- Human subject research

study findings have policy implications for improving clinical care and preventive interventions. As such, researchers should be honest with the beneficiaries and respondents, transparent about the findings and methodology, honest with other direct and indirect stakeholders, fulfill agreements and promises, and refrain from making false promises. In any scientific research, fraud, deceit, or misrepresentation are not acceptable and are strongly condemned by scientific committees, professionals, and the public.

20.5.2 Informed Consent

Informed consent is a process by which a subject voluntarily confirms his or her willingness to participate in research, after having been informed of all aspects of the research that are relevant to the subject's decision to participate. Informed consent is documented by means of a written, signed, and dated informed consent form.

Informed consent should always be taken and is needed because of: a) Greater patient safety and satisfaction, b) Attainment of higher ethical standards and organizational morale, c) Closer adherence to legal requirements and reduced risk of litigation, d) Increased level of institutional quality, and e) Potential time and money savings related to reduced litigation.

It is the obligation of researchers to provide relevant information about the research to study participants before obtaining their consent. Commonly, the information needed before a person decides whether to participate in the study includes:

- They need to know that it is research;
- They need to be told the purpose of the research;
- They need to know how long they will be expected to participate in the research;
- They need to know what you plan to do and what they are expected to do;
- They need to know which of the procedures are experimental, and if applicable how that might differ from anything they would undergo if they did not participate;
- They need to know potential risks or discomforts they may experience as a result of participating in the study;
- There is a need to address not only any physical risk to the participant but also any emotional or psychological risk or discomforts they may experience;
- They need to know what potential benefits they may receive by participating in the study without the overstating of any potential benefits;
- They need to know if there are any alternatives available to them should they choose not to participate;

- They need to know who is going to see the information they provide;
- If the study involves greater than minimal risk, the potential subject needs to know whether there will be any compensation and medical/psychological/social services available to them;
- They need to know that their participation is 100% voluntary. They will not be forced to participate and they will not be forced to stay in the study, should they want to withdraw at any time;
- They need to know who they can call or contact to ask questions about: a) Events that occur in the research; b) Their rights as participants in the research; and c) The person to contact if they become distressed, physically or emotionally injured; and
- Additional information that can be shared with the participants are: a) How many other people are participating in the study; and b) If new findings become available during the research that would impact their willingness to continue participation, you will share that information with them.

20.5.3 Consent Process

The consent process begins when you begin recruitment of subjects. Informed consent does not end with the signing of a document. The consent process is an ongoing, dynamic "conversation" with your subject to ensure: a) the person understands what is being asked of him/her; b) that the person has an opportunity to ask questions; and c) that the person truly wants to continue in the study.

20.5.4 Waiver of Consent

The IRB may waive the consent process if the following conditions exist: a) Retrospective studies, where the participants are de-identified or cannot be contacted; b) Research on anonymized biological samples/data; c) The rights and welfare of the subjects would not be adversely affected; d) Research on data available in the public domain; and e) Research during humanitarian emergencies and disasters, when the participant may not be in a position to give consent.

20.5.5 Who Can Give Consent?

Valid consent for participation in a study can be given by the participant themselves if they are an adult (over the age of 18) or if they have married, have been pregnant, or have graduated from a high school and the consent from another person is not necessary. The subject or subject's legally authorized representative can also give valid consent in exceptional circumstances such as: a) Children (parents give consent – child gives assent); c) Hearing or vision impaired; c) Individuals physically unable to sign; c) Prisoners; d) Cognitively impaired, mental disorders; and e) Illiterate persons (understands but does not read).

Consent should be taken (best practices) in a comfortable, private, and neutral setting, with or without family or friends, and with adequate time.

20.5.6 Problems with Consent Document

The consent form needs to be developed carefully so that no information, as discussed in Section 20.5.2, is omitted. The common problems with consent documents include:

- Information is not presented in terms the average person can understand (usually 8th grade level);
- Typographical or grammatical errors;
- All of the procedures are not included;
- The risks are not appropriately described;
- The benefits are overstated; and
- The person is not told that they are participating in research.

20.5.7 Assent

Assent means a child's affirmative agreement to participate in research, that is, to say "OK". Assent may be gained by talking with the child and supporting that talk with a written assent document appropriate to the child's age and comprehension level. In determining if children can give meaningful assent, the IRB will take into account the ages, maturity, and psychological state of the children, either individually or as a group, as it deems appropriate. For example, after 12 or 13 years of age, most children can adequately deal with abstract ideas.

20.5.8 Confidentiality

Confidentiality in the context of human research also refers to the investigator's agreement with participants, when applicable (i.e., through participants' informed consent), about how their identifiable private information will be handled, managed, and disseminated.

The IRB is responsible for evaluating proposed research to ensure adequate provisions to protect the privacy of participants and to maintain the confidentiality of data. Research involving human participants must include adequate provisions to maintain this confidentiality. Maintaining confidentiality requires safeguarding the information that an individual has disclosed in a relationship of trust and with the expectation that it will not be disclosed to others without permission, except in ways that are consistent with the original disclosure. Individuals may only be willing to share information for research purposes with an understanding that the information will remain protected from disclosure outside of the research setting or to unauthorized persons.

20.6 Research Ethical Committee

All studies involving humans as participants require a research ethics committee (REC) review. The principal investigator (or lead researcher on the study) is responsible for seeking this review. RECs protect research participants' rights, safety, dignity, and well-being. The name of the ethical approval board varies according to the organization. A few standard terms are Institutional Review Board (IRB), Ethics Review Committee (ERC), Research Review Committee (RRC), and Ethical Review Board (ERB).

20.6.1 Composition of an Institutional Review Board (IRB)

The federal policy requires that an IRB have at least five members: a chairperson, a scientific member, a nonscientific member, a lay person not affiliated with the institution, and a practitioner. The purpose of the IRB is to: a) assess the risks and benefits of the research; b) ensure that informed consent is obtained appropriately; c) verify that the recruitment methods/materials are not misleading; and d) ensure that the selection of subjects is equitable and justified.

The IRB must be sufficiently qualified through the experience and expertise of its members and the diversity of their backgrounds, including considerations of their racial and cultural heritage and their sensitivity to issues such as community attitudes, to promote respect for its advice and counsel in safeguarding the rights and welfare of human subjects. The composition of the board must provide the professional competence necessary to review research activities and be able to ascertain the acceptability of proposed research in terms of institutional commitments and regulations, applicable law, and standards of professional conduct and practice. No IRB may consist entirely of members of one profession. The board is not limited to five members and should be large enough to ensure adequate protection for vulnerable subjects. There are specific protections outlined by the Department of Education regarding handicapped children and mentally disabled persons [6]. The IRB may invite individuals who have competence in special topics to assist with review of projects outside the IRB members' expertise, but those invited individuals do not get to vote in IRB decisions. No IRB member may participate in the review of any project in which they have a conflicting interest, except to provide information. The membership of the IRB must be submitted to the Office for Protection from Research Risks and kept in the IRB's records. The membership list must include name, earned degrees, capacity, and experience sufficient to describe the member's contribution to IRB deliberations, and employment or other relationship with the institution or possible conflicts of interest [6]. In brief, the IRB should have:

- At least five members;
- At least one member with a scientific background;
- At least one member must be a non-scientist (this member must attend a meeting to achieve quorum);
- At least one non-affiliated member (not affiliated with the institution);
- Members should have expertise in the research that will be reviewed; and
- A lawyer.

20.7 Common Research Misconducts

Research ethics ensure the safety of study subjects as well as the researcher. The research ethics also provide the researcher with a sense of responsibility. Therefore, all researchers must follow ethical guidelines. Here are some standard unethical practices every researcher must avoid: a) Data manipulation, including falsification and omission; b) Discussing confidential data with colleagues; c) Failing to keep good research records; d) Making a significant variation from the research protocol approved by ERC and SRC without permission; e) Not reporting an adverse event; f) Exposing research participants to biological risks; g) Image manipulation; and h) Plagiarism.

Finally, if research is based on a robust design and safely, ethically, and properly done, it can benefit all. Professional codes, laws, regulations, and ethical committees can provide guidance, but the ultimate determinant rests with the researcher's values and moral principles.

References

1. Mandal J, Acharya S, Parija SC. Ethics in human research. *Trop Parasitol.* 2011;1(1):2–3. Available from: www.ncbi.nlm.nih.gov/pmc/articles/PMC 3593469/#:~:text=

2. Rice TW. The historical, ethical, and legal background of human-subjects research. *Respir Care*. 2008;53(10):1325–9. Available from: https://pubmed. ncbi.nlm.nih.gov/18811995

3. University of Nevada. History of Research Ethics. Available from: www. unlv.edu/research/ORI-HSR/history-ethics

4. Komesaroff P, Dodds SM, McNeill P, Skene L, Thomson C. *Human Research Ethics Handbook: Commentary on the National Statement on Ethical Conduct in Research Involving Humans*; 2002. Available from: http://ecite.utas.edu. au/90916

5. US department of health and human services. The Belmont Report; 2023. Available from: www.hhs.gov/ohrp/regulations-and-policy/belmont-rep ort/index.html

6. Enfield KB, Truwit JD. The purpose, composition, and function of an institutional review board: Balancing priorities. *Respir Care*. 2008 Oct;53(10):1330–6. PubMed PMID: 18811996.

Index